Psychiatric Aspects of Reproductive Technology

ISSUES IN
PSYCHIATRY

Joseph D. Bloom, M.D.
Series Editor

Psychiatric Aspects of Reproductive Technology

Edited by

Nada L. Stotland, M.D.

Associate Professor of Clinical Psychiatry and Clinical Obstetrics and Gynecology, and Psychiatric Liaison and Consultant to Obstetrics and Gynecology, The University of Chicago, Chicago, Illinois

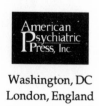

American Psychiatric Press, Inc

Washington, DC
London, England

Copyright 1990 American Psychiatric Press, Inc.
ALL RIGHTS RESERVED
Manufactured in the United States of America
First Edition
90 91 92 93 4 3 2 1

American Psychiatric Press, Inc.
1400 K Street, N.W., Washington, DC 20005

The paper used in this publication meets the minimum requirements of the American National Standard for Information Sciences—Permanence of Paper for Printed Library Materials, ANSI Z39.48-1984. ∞

Library of Congress Cataloging-in-Publication Data

Psychiatric aspects of reproductive technology / edited by Nada L. Stotland.
     p.   cm.—(Issues in psychiatry)
  Includes bibliographical references.
  ISBN 0-88048-316-4 (alk. paper)
    1. Human reproductive technology—Psychological aspects.
I. Stotland, Nada Logan.
  [DNLM: 1. Reproduction Technics—psychology. WQ 205 P974]
  RG133.5.P78 1990
  616.6'92'0019—dc20
  DLC
  for Library of Congress
                                    90-266
                                    CIP

British Library Cataloguing in Publication Data

A CIP record is available from the British Library.

To Harold

Contents

Contributors

Roberta J. Apfel, M.D., M.P.H.
Associate Professor of Clinical Psychiatry, Harvard University Medical School, Boston, Massachusetts

Colleen K. Connell, J.D.
Director and Legal Counsel for the Reproductive Rights Project of the American Civil Liberties Union of Illinois

Christine L. Cook, M.D.
Associate Professor, Department of Obstetrics and Gynecology, University of Louisville, Louisville, Kentucky

Leah J. Dickstein, M.D.
Professor, Department of Psychiatry and Behavioral Sciences, and Associate Dean for Faculty and Student Advocacy, University of Louisville School of Medicine, Louisville, Kentucky

Jennifer Downey, M.D.
Assistant Clinical Professor of Psychiatry, New York State Psychiatric Institute and Department of Psychiatry, Columbia University College of Physicians and Surgeons, New York, New York

Susan M. Fisher, M.D.
Clinical Associate Professor, Department of Psychiatry, University of Chicago, Chicago, Illinois

Michelle Harrison, M.D.
Assistant Professor of Psychiatry, University of Pittsburgh, Western Psychiatric Institute and Clinic, Pittsburgh, Pennsylvania

John D. Lantos, M.D.
Assistant Professor of Pediatrics and Assistant Director, Center for Clinical Medical Ethics, University of Chicago Pritzker School of Medicine, Chicago, Illinois

Cheryl F. McCartney, M.D.
Associate Professor of Psychiatry and Adjunctive Associate Professor of Obstetrics and Gynecology, University of North Carolina School of Medicine, Chapel Hill, North Carolina

Mary McKinney, M.A.
Doctoral Candidate, Department of Psychology, City College of New York, New York, New York

Michael F. Myers, M.D., F.R.C.P.(C)
Coordinator of Medical Student Interns, Department of Psychiatry, University Hosptial—Shaughnessy Site, and Clinical Professor, Department of Psychiatry, The University of British Columbia, Vancouver, British Columbia

Malkah T. Notman, M.D.
Training and Supervising Psychoanalyst, Boston Psychoanalytic Society and Institute, and Clinical Professor of Psychiatry, Harvard University Medical School, Boston, Massachusetts

Miriam B. Rosenthal, M.D.
Associate Professor, Psychiatry and Reproductive Biology, Case Western Reserve University, MacDonald Hospital for Women, Cleveland, Ohio

Nada L. Stotland, M.D.
Associate Professor of Clinical Psychiatry and Clinical Obstetrics and Gynecology, and Psychiatric Liaison and Consultant to Obstetrics and Gynecology, The University of Chicago, Chicago, Illinois

Cicilia Y. Wada, Ph.D.
Biostatistician, Campinas University, Campinas, Brazil

Acknowledgments

I would like to thank Carol Nadelson for her ideas and support. Carol Magnussen's organization, persistence, and hard work were essential to the completion of the project. Joseph Bloom inspired me with enthusiasm and confidence and followed through with careful readings and thoughtful suggestions.

Chapter 1

Introduction and Overview

Nada L. Stotland, M.D.

Formal American Psychiatric Association (APA) focus on psychiatric issues in reproductive technologies began in the APA Committee on
Women, which proposed a task force to examine and address these issues
in June of 1987. Controversial court cases involving new reproductive styles,
notably the so-called surrogate mother custody case of Mary Beth Whitehead
and the Sterns, had alerted the public and the psychiatric community to the
increasing frequency of nontraditional methods of reproduction and to their
emotional complications and central psychological unknowns. In some cases,
including this one, psychiatrists had actually testified as expert witnesses.
Psychologists had participated in the screening process as a result of which
Ms. Whitehead was selected by the Sterns to conceive, bear, and relinquish
custody of a child biologically fathered by Mr. Stern.

A 1-day meeting sponsored by the APA in September of 1987 brought
together representatives of many components of the APA, including
research; law; governmental relations; children, adolescents, and families;
public affairs; and women. Representatives of the American College of Obstetricians and Gynecologists also participated and submitted relevant docu-
ments. After hearing and discussing the perspectives of these participants,
the group decided unanimously to recommend to the Board of Trustees that
the APA appoint a task force to address psychiatric aspects of new reproductive technologies from an organizational and operational standpoint. This
volume will address the need for a reference work for psychiatric clinicians,
educators, and trainees, taking a multidisciplinary informational standpoint.

This chapter describes the sociohistorical context out of which arose a need
for this volume, drawing on the more extensive treatments of the currently
relevant issues to be found in the ensuing chapters. Recent technologic
developments are synergistic with people's expectation that medical/tech-

nical solutions to any physiologic problem can and must be found. Both of these affect and are affected by the traditional and changing psychology of reproduction for women and for men, and the traditional and evolving social conditions in which people contemplate and experience parenthood. Psychological, sociological, medical, and technological pressures converge to produce a tremendous thrust toward the use of new methods of conception.

Lesson From History: DES

Possibly the long-term effects of past attempts at constructive reproductive interventions, such as the use of diethylstilbestrol (DES) in pregnancy, offer lessons that have not been applied (Apfel and Fisher 1984). DES was a treatment first prescribed for so-called habitual aborters—women who had spontaneously miscarried in two or more previous pregnancies. It was hypothesized that hormone deficiency was the cause of the miscarriage, and exogenous hormone administration the remedy. A fervent group of medical believers promulgated and popularized the treatment, and the indications for its use in some settings widened to include all pregnant women.

Both the faith of the believers and the widespread prescriptions outlived what positive medical evidence there had been. They persisted even when it was clear that there was no evidence of benefit and despite concern about possible long-term effects. Then, otherwise rare reproductive tract malignancies and anomalies began to surface in the children who had been exposed to DES in utero. The mothers who had been willing and eager to do anything to maintain and strengthen their unborn children had unwittingly been a party to hurting them.

Not only have the families suffered from the defects and malignancies themselves, but also the nature of the injury compromises and complicates the mother-child relationship. The children's reproductive function has been hampered by their mothers' efforts to improve their own. Their trust in mother's nurture, and mother's self-esteem in her parental role, are complementarily threatened.

Similarly, the relationships between mothers and/or children affected by DES and the medical community are more or less permanently undermined. DES was suggested and prescribed by doctors. In some cases, those doctors and the institutions in which the women were treated have neglected or refused to locate, counsel, evaluate, and treat them and their children despite the clear evidence that they are at risk. Even in cases where follow-up has been good, and where women understand intellectually that the involved physicians were making a sincere attempt to help them with DES, basic trust was betrayed at a deeper, psychological level. The powerful expert, the caretaker, has not only failed to help, but has caused harm. The harm is manifested in the very organs and functions that the treatment was meant to foster: the reproductive capacity that is such a private and precious part of personal and gender identity.

For identified children at risk, gynecologic surveillance begins around puberty—just when mother, and sometimes the gynecologist, is normally called on to affirm the adolescent's health and gender adequacy while respecting developmental needs of adolescents.

There are a number of relevant issues for psychiatrists involved with the new reproductive technologies. It is important to understand these dynamics of DES-affected patients, the risks they face, the situation out of which they arose, and the evaluations and treatment they undergo. In addition, psychiatrists and patients now contemplating reproductive interventions may view this as a cautionary tale. When present with considerable anxiety, is this normal or neurotic?

Babies conceived by in vitro fertilization and other techniques appear grossly normal at birth and in early childhood. But we do not yet know the long-term effects of the many hormonal and surgical components of some of the new means of procreation. Although efforts are made to assess the possible negative effects of new procedures, controlled studies on human subjects are not ethical. Many health care professionals, in their eagerness to offer instrumental relief for human suffering and/or to exercise scientific control over a fantastically complicated physiologic process, do not focus on these unknowns. Many people who wish to become parents (or, in the case of some technologies, not to become parents) do not consider them. What constitutes informed consent for these patients? Difficult questions exist for the psychiatrist in counseling for decision making, gatekeeping, and/or therapeutic work with those involved.

Recent Controversies: So-Called Surrogacy as a Case in Point

Clearly, dynamic issues overlap and interact with the ethical and legal issues that have come into focus as a result of new reproductive practices. So-called surrogate mother cases are a poignant example in our more recent history (American Fertility Society Committee on Ethics 1986). One case in particular has been widely publicized. Not only have reports of the facts been chronicled in sometimes doubtful detail, and legal issues been debated with varying degrees of depth and accuracy, but a television movie depicting the circumstances has already been aired.

The Sterns were a childless couple. Mr. Stern, a biochemist, particularly wanted to have biological children because many of his relatives had perished during World War II. Mrs. Stern, a pediatrician, had diagnosed herself as a victim of multiple sclerosis, and therefore at risk of exacerbation from pregnancy. A volunteer, Mrs. Mary Beth Whitehead, was found, psychologically evaluated, and paid $10,000 under a contractual arrangement to undergo artificial insemination by Mr. Stern's sperm and bear a child whose custody she would relinquish to the Sterns. After the child was born and relinquished, Mrs. Whitehead changed her mind, took her daughter, and defied a court order to return her. After considerable litigation, the child now (January 1989) resides with the Sterns and sees her biological mother on weekends.

While some observers, including the judge who first heard the Whitehead-Stern case, construed the case as an issue of contract law, many others conceptualized the problem in psychological and psychiatric terms. Surely a simple contract dispute would not have generated so much affect and attention. What was Mrs. Whitehead's state of mental health—normality or illness, fragility, or deviance? By what standards and which professionals could it best be evaluated? Was it relevant? What outcome would be in the best interest of the child? Should the child's best interest be construed in terms of financial comfort and intellectual advantages, or in terms of psychological attachment and identity?

As we have seen, in the larger context of reproductive technologies, complex legal, ethical, religious, and social questions are added to the psychological ones with which psychiatrists generally deal. In fact, in each case, and for each technology, the participants, public representatives, and clinicians must decide how to construe the issues—whether as case studies or moral dilemmas, breaches of contract or sins. Decisions such as these are often made by assumption, on the basis of the context: legal constructions in the courts, pathologic diagnoses in the clinical setting, moral transgressions in the confessional.

Much conflict and bewilderment arise from the many situations where there is a poor fit between context and approach. Do psychiatrists belong in courts of law? Do lawyers belong in custody decisions? Should reproductive technologists make decisions about the management of the conceptus?

What are the social implications of so-called surrogacy? Autonomy is a major concern. Some argue that women have a right to use, enjoy, and profit from their bodies as they see fit. Others see surrogacy as the exploitation of emotionally and financially vulnerable women as genetic and gestational objects for wealthier and more sophisticated couples. The impact on the other children of the woman who conceives, gestates, and gives up an infant is another clinical and ethical issue.

Legislation has been introduced in a number of states to regulate surrogacy and other reproductive variations. Some proposed statutes would limit or ban it; others would reinforce contract provisions. Some mandate mental health involvement of one sort or another. This, too, raises an ethical question. Perhaps all persons in the throes of these difficult decisions and procedures should have access to psychotherapeutic assessment, support, and guidance. Should they be required? Who is best qualified to provide them? Persons who do not require technological assistance are free to become parents without the involvement of mental health professionals . 1979).

Definitions

What are the new reproductive technologies? The term *new reproductive technologies* was chosen for this volume not because of its precise medical accuracy, but because it evokes the dilemmas the volume addresses (Kieffer 1979). As used herein, it includes both techniques that require the most delicate hormonal and surgical manipulations, and that were not possible a few years ago, and simpler procedures that raise some of the same questions. The techniques are discussed, from the viewpoint of the practicing gynecologist, elsewhere (Cook, Chapter 5, this volume).

Reproductive technologies fall into four main categories: in vitro fertilization; hormone manipulation, often to stimulate ovulation; surgery; and monitoring technologies. In vitro fertilization is used for women whose infertility is due to blockage or nonfunction of the fallopian tubes, whereas the ovaries and uterus are normal. Menstrual cycles are hormonally controlled so that several ova "ripen" at once, at a time when the laboratory, technologists, and the male partner are available. The ova are identified and located by ultrasound, surgically "harvested," and fertilized with semen the partner obtains by masturbating. The woman is hormonally prepared for implantation, and when one or more embryos are ready for this stage, they are transferred from the laboratory vessel into the reproductive tract.

The procedure involves significant discomfort, expense, inconvenience, and risk of failure. Prospective parents become attached to the fertilized eggs, some of which may be frozen for use in subsequent attempts. (Siblings born some years apart may have been conceived at the same time.) Disposition of these human embryos has been a matter of considerable ethical and legal dispute. Related technologies involve donor oocytes, donor embryos, and intrafallopian gamete transfer. A woman giving birth to a child may not be its genetic mother; her sexual partner or husband may not be its genetic father (Christie and Pawson 1987).

Ovulation-stimulating drugs are a related category of infertility treatment. The "old" generation of drugs has been supplemented by a new one. As is the case with in vitro fertilization, indications for this management have evolved and broadened over recent years. Surgical techniques for the diagnosis and management of reproductive problems have proliferated and been increasingly refined. Many women will experience laparoscopies and endoscopies during which their reproductive structures can be directly scrutinized. Once mysterious and inaccessible organs are exposed and often photographed, and then described to the anxious patients. Cautery, laser ablation, and coagulation procedures can lyse adhesions and minimize endometriosis.

Sequential, microsurgical reconstructions can restore the potency and physiologic function of damaged fallopian tubes.

Some centers include psychological, psychiatric, or other mental health screening and/or counseling as part of these processes; others do not. There are no general guidelines either for the use of mental health services or for admission to, and termination of, any of these attempts at treatment. This issue will be discussed further in this and the ensuing chapters of this volume.

Last, a new array of technologies are available for monitoring the status of reproductive events. There are home tests for ovulation and pregnancy and radioimmune assays for reproductive hormones. Ultrasound is used to diagnose defects in reproductive organs or developing fetuses, and as a necessary component of other technologies, as in the detection of ovulation in preparation for in vitro fertilization or the location of the placenta and fetus during amniocentesis. Many obstetricians consider ultrasound monitoring to be an important tool in the routine prenatal care of low-risk women. Prospective parents' experience of pregnancy and attachment to the fetus is profoundly affected by the image they can observe on the screen from very early in gestation.

The substitution of a "handmaiden" for a wife for the purpose of reproduction in the male family line is described the Bible. Artificial insemination can be performed by amateurs using extremely primitive equipment. But the popularization of noncoital reproduction, especially between nonmarital partners, has evoked in many individuals and social institutions the sense that fundamental elements of our developmental psychologies and social organization, factors that were considered and experienced as "givens," are being challenged.

The Role of the Psychiatrist

These effects of reproductive technologies stimulate psychiatrists in particular to reconsider traditional assumptions. Is the Oedipus complex a universal product of a particular family structure? How vital is the need for a male, or a second parent, in normal child development? Is the desire for biological offspring a normal, universal given, or a narcissistic self-indulgence? Do biological relations between parent and child increase healthy connectedness, or foster neurotic or at least unrealistic expectations and conflicts (Williams 1986)?

We lack the follow-up data on which we might predicate regulations, priorities, and psychiatric practice (Daniluk et al. 1985). But psychiatrists have been, will be, and probably should be called on to play major roles in the arena of reproductive technology. There are several reasons. Psychiatrists have generations of experience with human dynamics and behaviors to bring to bear on regulations, priorities, and clinical situations. Patients and professionals contemplating the use of reproductive technologies need flexible guidelines and advice on the issues of entry decision making; relationships between patients, doctors, and others involved, such as program coordinators and technicians; informed consent; pacing and goal setting; terminating treatment; and making decisions about childlessness or adoption (Rosenfeld and Mitchell 1979).

Psychiatrists are both physicians and mental health professionals; this combination makes psychiatrists particularly useful in understanding medical procedures and translating them into human terms. We can apply our awareness that human behaviors and desires derive from complex layers of motivations, conflicts, and fears. We are expert in communication skills and mediation. We have considerable knowledge and sophistication in research on similar issues and can foster the application of this knowledge to the formulation of research questions and the development of the research projects so desperately needed in these areas (Mazor 1984).

This volume is intended to prepare the interested psychiatric generalist or subspecialist to address this range of psychiatric roles related to reproductive technologies. New developments act on a substrate of cultural and psychological correlates and traditions, so we begin with a review of the psychology of women with respect to reproduction. Feminist scholarship and politics highlight two somewhat paradoxically opposed facets of the current state of knowledge.

On the one hand, it can be argued that both the biological and psychological aspects of female reproduction have been comparatively ignored in the research literature (Williams 1983). Biopsychological changes correlated with the menstrual cycle, pregnancy, birth, lactation, and menopause have been sparsely studied. Important psychiatric aspects of these reproductive events have not been addressed. For example, in studies of psychoactive drugs, both cyclic and reproductive life-cycle changes and the possibility of pregnancy have been regarded as confounding variables and/or sources of serious legal liability, so that males tend to be the only subjects. Dispensing literature includes a warning that the drug's safety during pregnancy and lactation has not been established, and no other information about effects linked to human reproductive variables is available.

In research on other psychiatric and psychological issues, reproductive life-cycle factors have been almost universally overlooked (Stotland 1988). For example, recent attempts to clarify the relationship between parturition and psychiatric illness are hampered by the fact that psychiatric hospital records often do not indicate whether or not a woman had delivered in the months preceding admission. The same is true of gynecologic complications and procedures, such as hysterectomy, miscarriage, and elective abortion. The lack of scientific attention to these issues deprives clinicians, who share this cultural inattention, of a knowledge base that would inform diagnostic and therapeutic efforts.

On the other hand, attention directed to the psychobehavioral correlates of reproductive events can reinforce culturally based notions that women's physiology is incapacitating, and that, therefore, women are less suited than men to make significant decisions and occupy positions of responsibility. This debate was joined with considerable passion, evoked formidable debate, and required skillful arbitration when a diagnostic category, informally called premenstrual syndrome and formalized as periluteal phase dysphoric disorder, was proposed for the revision of the third edition of the *Diagnostic and Statistical Manual of Mental Disorders* (American Psychiatric Association 1987). A compromise was struck; the proposed diagnosis, along with others that were of clinical and research interest but were insufficiently substantiated and/or socially problematic, was described in a differentiated appendix, to be used for research purposes (American Psychiatric Association 1987). It is clear to involved clinicians that reproductive changes and milestones are an important element in women's psychological development, dynamics, and functioning. Women bring to the situations occasioning the use of reproductive technology, and to the technologic interventions themselves, both these givens and their acute reactions to medical complications and the interaction with the health care system. Psychiatrists bring scientific knowledge, clinical skills, and their own traditions and prejudices.

The Social Context

Yet another major element in the interplay between women's reproductive psychology and reproductive technology is changes in social attitudes and policies concerning procreation (Riech 1978). Women with active career ambitions and pursuits tend to postpone childbearing and are therefore at increased risk of infertility (Lidz 1978). These same women have, as important components of their character structures and life histories, the conviction that all aims can be achieved and all obstacles overcome by a combination of intelligence, knowledge, innovation, persistence, and financial outlay. These are the very factors offered as solutions to fertility problems, and accepted as assets in potential patients, by the practitioners of reproductive technologies.

While some women postpone having children, they are under several constraints to produce them expeditiously when they eventually decide to do so (Ziman-Tobin 1986). Their own parents will have waited, with whatever degree of impatience, for what has been perceived as an extended period of time for grandchildren. Their remaining years of potential fertility and of energy for child rearing are limited. Their careers may demand that conception be carefully timed so as not to interfere with professional obligations. All these pressures combine with their frustrated parental longings to produce an urgency that has a potent emotional effect on the people who control, facilitate, and provide reproductive technology (Seastrunk et al. 1984).

Although hard data have not been gathered, it seems fairly clear that social attitudes toward children conceived and born of nonmarital and/or noncoital circumstances, and their families, are more accepting than in centuries, decades, years, perhaps even months, past. "Society" may even be more accepting than the parents themselves. For example, most parents who conceive by artificial donor insemination have conflicts over whether to inform family, friends, or the children so conceived (Notman 1984).

It may be that newspaper headlines and television reports are novelties, and that unorthodox reproductive techniques, if revealed, do skew the relationships between families using them and significant others. But reluctance to parent a child of another color, race, or ethnic background may underlie the decision of some prospective parents to use reproductive technologies rather than adopt a child. There is a shortage of healthy, white newborns available for adoption. Many couples desiring children want children both as much like themselves and as unlikely to attract attention as possible. In addition, media explanations and exposure of reproductive technologies combine with increased societal openness about sex and reproduction (which has been given further impetus by the problem of acquired immunodeficiency syndrome) to facilitate public acceptance of technologically achieved conceptions and the families created by them.

With respect to the relationship between women and health care providers, another paradox has arisen. Some women are skeptical or frankly hostile about paternalistic styles of medical care, but still need reassurance and direction when under the stress of infertility, labor, or surgery. Psychiatrists can help reproductive care providers deal with the fact that patients' attitudes are sometimes state-dependent rather than trait-dependent. Decisions about technologic interventions are often made under the conditions just described, rather than as a result of dispassionate reason. Psychiatrists can help infertile couples review their values and goals, as well as the pressures of the situation, to improve the experience and quality of decision making (Seibel and Taymor 1982). Health care providers must decide whether, and at what point, continued endeavors and interventions are psychiatrically, as well as medically, indicated.

These dilemmas highlight a fascinating imponderable: under what circumstances, for what reasons, and at what cost, pain, and risk is it psychiatrically healthy or unhealthy to attempt to conceive? We have not had to consider this question in general, since sufficient numbers of babies are born to maintain and increase the population. The issue does come up with regard to subpopulations or individual patients who conceive and deliver under conditions that are personally and/or socially disadvantageous, such as patients in adolescence or with schizophrenia, interfering with effective parenting (Riech 1978).

The Psychological Context: Fertility and Infertility

The major population facing the question of how much time, energy, affect, physical discomfort and risk, and money reproduction is worth is the infertile population, estimated at 10% of United States couples (Kraft et al. 1980). While techniques such as chorionic villi sampling, ultrasound surveillance of low-risk pregnancies, and fetal monitoring are relatively new reproductive technologies affecting many patients, the thrust of the interest and controversy centers on techniques used for those who are reproductively compromised in some way. These patients are making their treatment decisions, undergoing the procedures, and parenting the resulting children, if any, in psychological circumstances colored by that infertility.

Underlying the psychological meanings of infertility is the significant place of fertility in human psychodynamics and development (Mazor 1984). For women especially, reproductive events are psychosocial milestones around which the course of life is fantasized, planned, and experienced. The possibility of future parenthood is important to children of both sexes from a very early age onward. Traditionally in our society, motherhood was to girls' futures what jobs were to boys. The association of puberty with the capacity to conceive seems more integral to young women's education and experience. Planning for parenthood is more central to women's lives than to men's for three reasons: the physical demands and risks of childbearing affect only women, women continue to assume the overwhelming share of child-rearing obligations, and women's fertility ends with menopause.

Fertility is and becomes very important to men as well. It signifies not only the capacity for procreation, with the gratification of parenting and continuing the family line and name, but also virility. Men who discover that they have impaired fertility are at risk for impotence (Berger 1980). Both members of an infertile couple experience decreased self-esteem. Marital stress may be so severe as to result in divorce. Men and women have demonstrably different styles of dealing with infertility; men are secretive, whereas women feel a need to share feelings and narratives with others (McCartney and Wada, Chapter 11, this volume). The effort to conceive and the fertility workup and treatment transform the experience of the sexual act from one of spontaneity and affection into one of rigid schedules and goal directedness. Intense attention of the couple is focused on bodily functions and cycles.

Reproductive interventions in the context of infertility raise several questions for the psychiatrist. Has the response to reproductive incompetence been worked through? Will the use of technology foster psychological adaptation or postpone or obstruct the acceptance of the problem? What is the state of the relationship between the fertile and infertile partner? Are they equally committed to the treatment? Is the fertile partner resentful? Is the infertile partner denigrated? How may their reproductive problem affect their ability to foster a healthy gender identity and sexual attitudes in any children they may have? Is the search for technologic assistance a symptom of inability to accept their reproductive state? How will they manage if the treatment is unsuccessful?

Single, or unpartnered, women wishing to conceive face considerable prejudice and, often, obstacles, when they seek medical help. If they are infertile, they must deal with their feelings and treatments alone. Fertile women in increasing numbers wish to conceive without what they perceive as the encumbrance of a relationship with a man in the absence of a mutual commitment to each other and to parenthood. They seek artificial insemination to avoid this complication and the necessity to have intercourse simply to conceive. They expect that the medical facility will screen the sperm donors. Some simply want to be assured that the biological father is healthy and free of known genetic disorders; others arrange to be inseminated with sperm of men with chosen traits. There is a sperm bank for Nobel Prize winners. Women can choose donors by intelligence quotient, job field, appearance, and/or hobbies. Presumably these choices indicate something of their wishes and fantasies for their offspring; no systematic follow-up has been performed to determine whether the children have the desired traits or how these expectations affect them.

Conclusions: Directions

In all of the foregoing, the need for research has been apparent and significant. The identification of problems must proceed and coincide with the search for answers. Psychiatrists and other mental health professionals have been and should be involved in the formulation of these research questions and the performance of the research itself. They have relevant expertise to offer the legislatures and the courts as they attempt to make sense of and regularize reproductive technology practice for the good of society. They can collaborate with the reproductive technologists who select, prepare, and treat patients. Practicing psychiatric clinicians may use this volume to understand and work with patients affected by these profound changes and opportunities in human reproduction.

References

American Fertility Society Committee on Ethics: Ethical considerations   of the new reproductive technologies. Fertil Steril 46 (Suppl 1), no 3, 1986

American Psychiatric Association: Diagnostic and Statistical Manual of Mental Disorders, 3rd Edition, Revised. Washington, DC, American Psychiatric Association, 1987

Apfel RJ, Fisher SM: To Do No Harm: DES and the Dilemmas of Modern Medicine. New Haven, CT, Yale University Press, 1984

Berger DM: Couples' reactions to male infertility and donor insemination. Am J Psychiatry 137:1047–1049, 1980

Christie GL, Pawson ME: The psychological and social management of the infertile couple, in The Infertile Couple. Edited by Pepperell RJ, Hudson B, Wood C. New York, Churchill Livingstone, 1987, pp 35–50

Daniluk J, Leader A, Taylor PJ: The psychological sequelae of infertility, in The Psychiatric Implications of Menstruation. Edited by Gold JH. Washington, DC, American Psychiatric Press, 1985, pp 75–85

Kieffer G: Reproductive technologies: a sampler of issues, in Bioethics: A Textbook of Issues. Reading, MA, Menlo Park, CA, 1979, pp 47–63

Kraft AD, Palombo J, Mitchell D, et al: The Psychological Dimensions of Infertility. Am J Orthopsychiatry 50:618–628, 1980

Lidz RW: Conflicts between fertility and infertility, in The Women Patient: Medical and Psychological Interfaces, Vol 1: Sexual and Reproductive Aspects of Women's Health Care. Edited by Notman MT, Nadelson CC. New York, Plenum, 1978, pp 121–129

Mazor MD: Emotional reactions to infertility, in Infertility: Medical, Emotional, and Social Considerations. Edited by Mazor MD, Simons HF. New York, Human Sciences Press, 1984

Notman MT: Psychological aspects of artificial donor insemination, in Infertility: Medical, Emotional, and Social Considerations. Edited by Mazor MD, Simons HF. New York, Human Sciences Press, 1984

Riech PA: Historical understanding of contraception, in The Woman Patient, Medical and Psychological Interfaces, Vol 1. Edited by Notman MT, Nadelson CC. New York, Plenum, 1978, pp 215–241

Rosenfeld DL, Mitchell E: Treating the emotional aspects of infertility: counseling services in an infertility clinic. Am J Obstet Gynecol 136:177–180, 1979

Seastrunk JW, de Benkemery T, Adelsberg B, et al: Psychological evaluation of couples in an impatient reproductive biology unit. Fertil Steril 41:965, 1984

Seibel MM, Taymor ML: Emotional aspects of infertility. Fertil Steril 37:137–145, 1982

Stotland NL: Social Change and Women's Reproductive Health Care. New York, Praeger, 1988

Williams JH: Psychology of Women: Behavior in a Biosocial Context. New York, WW Norton, 1983

Williams SL: Reproductive motivations and contemporary feminine development, in The Psychology of Today's Woman: New Psychoanalytic Visions. Edited by Bernay T, Cantor DW. Hillsdale, NJ, Analytic Press, 1986, pp 68–79

Ziman-Tobin P: Childless women approaching midlife: issues in psychoanalytic treatment, in The Psychology of Today's Woman: New Psychoanalytic Visions. Edited by Bernay T, Cantor DW. Hillsdale, NJ, Analytic Press, 1986, pp 81–95

Chapter 2

Reproduction and Pregnancy: A Psychodynamic Developmental Perspective

Malkah T. Notman, M.D.

Fertility is revered in almost all cultures, and pregnancy is a milestone in adult development. It is the bridge between generations, rich in symbolism and central in human experience. For a woman, the knowledge that she is able to bear children has been critical in the development of her sense of femininity, gender identity, and self-esteem, even if she chooses not to have children as an adult. The awareness of her reproductive potential is part of her self-image.

The social changes of the past two decades have also brought shifts in family patterns and life-styles. With more effective control of contraception possible, and many more women working, women have been seeking fulfillment in terms other than a career of motherhood. Having a baby, although pivotal psychologically and physically, may not provide the only way to attain adulthood and status as a woman. Many women have been delaying pregnancy. Some have encountered fertility problems; others become mothers at a point in their own lives when individuation, ego development, and consolidation of self have progressed to a different level than for a younger woman. The effects of the life stage of the individual on the significance and course of the pregnancy have not been fully studied.

There appears to be new interest in the psychodynamic aspects of pregnancy. In the psychoanalytic literature, there was an early focus on the symbolic meaning of a pregnancy but not on the actual experience for the woman until the 1940s (Deutsch 1944, 1945) and 1950s (Benedek and Rubenstein 1952).

13

In this chapter I present an overview of psychodynamic psychoanalytic concepts about reproductive motivation and a brief review of concepts of femininity as the preparation for becoming pregnant. Then the developmental function that pregnancy has for a woman will be discussed.

Early Psychoanalytic Views

Pregnancy was not an important focus for Freud, nor the early psychoanalysts. It is now a well-known critique that Freud derived his views about female psychology and sexuality from theories about men and male sexuality. He believed that early sexuality was originally masculine: "The sexuality of little girls is of a wholly masculine character" (Freud 1905, p. 219). The little girl was "really" castrated, and the baby she came to want was the symbolic substitution for the "missing" penis.

Freud saw the female psyche as enigmatic. He considered the little girl to be "masculine" for the first few years of her life—or at any rate not different from a little boy. After feeling disappointed in her mother, who she felt had failed to give her a penis, and whom she additionally devalued as having no penis herself, she turned to her father. This turning to the father follows the girl's discovery of the anatomic differences between the sexes and her "narcissistic humiliation." Unable to compete with boys, the girl "gives up her wish for a penis and puts in place of it a wish for a child, and with that purpose in view she takes her father as a love object" (Freud 1925, p. 256; also see Freud 1932). These formulations, supported by clinical observations of adults interpreted within this framework, formed the basis for understanding the nature of the little girl's wish for a child as a symbolic substitute for the penis she does not have. In this reasoning, the wish for a baby is not really the same as a wish for a pregnancy, or a wish to be a mother. Nor was it connected with the capacity for motherliness in the sense of the ability to relate to a child as a separate person, and to understand and meet a child's needs. Procreation as a wider goal for either women or men was not explicitly or directly explored.

The sources of procreative wishes or drives were sought in instinctual drives and biological forces. In humans, the biological components of the wish to reproduce have been difficult to define, since instinctual life is overlaid by many learned responses and by the impact of socialization. In animals, one can trace certain sexual behaviors as responses to particular hormonal variations; in humans, this is only partially established.

The wish for pregnancy and for a child can be considered part of this larger wish to procreate that is universal. Parenthood itself, involving the caring and nurturing relationship with a child, was not a central concern to early psychoanalytic writers. Parenthood calls on early affects, physical experiences of the parent when he or she was a child (Sadow 1984), as well as on identifications from all one's earlier life. It has been considered a developmental process (Benedek 1974, quoted in Parens 1975; Schwartz 1984) or phase (Benedek 1959) that enables the person to assume adult roles and fulfill adult societal expectations. One element of the wish to procreate is, therefore, to be an adult like one's parents. This is true even if the actual process of becoming mature is short-circuited, as is often the case in teenage pregnancy. In his concept of generativity, Erikson (1963) described "the concern in establishing and guiding the next generation" (p. 267), although he distinguished generativity from actual procreation and included creativity in this concept. Becoming a parent provides a small piece of immortality, an extension into the future, and offers the illusion of being godlike in the creation of life.

Psychoanalytic interest in motherhood then began to include actual maternal experiences and attitudes. Deutsch (1945) wrote about the "active ingredients" of the "joys of motherhood"; she described this form of activity (as compared to the passivity that was considered part of the nature of femininity) as an aspect of the maternal function that was not "of an aggressive masculine character" but "closest to the phylogenetic and the instinctual" (p. 127). She also believed that some unconscious hostility to the fetus characterized almost every pregnant woman, an idea that did not gain recognition in the then prevalent obstetrical view of pregnancy as a blissful state.

Benedek (1959) also was interested in the psychobiology of pregnancy. She described pregnancy as a "critical phase" in the life of a woman. Benedek and Rubenstein (1952) studied the affective correlates of the cyclic endocrine changes of the menstrual cycle as measured with the techniques available at the time. Their observations led them to hypothesize different emotional manifestations of different phases of the menstrual cycle. Motherhood, in Benedek's (1970) view, is not secondary or a substitute for the missing penis, but is the "manifestation of the all-pervading instinct for survival in the child that is the primary organizer of the woman's sexual drive, and by this also of her personality" (p. 139). She thought that pregnancy revived developmental conflicts that influenced women's feelings about motherhood and their attitudes toward their children.

Benedek (1970) traced the changes in narcissism during the course of the pregnancy, as did Deutsch (1944, 1945). In her conceptualization of motherliness as arising in part from the response to the child and as the organizer of a woman's sexual drive, Benedek anticipated more recent writers, who have stressed the nonsubstitutive nature of the wish for a child, and see it as a primary part of feminine orientation and fulfillment (Chasseguet-Smirgel 1970; Kestenberg 1976; Stoller 1976).

Although Benedek (1970) and others saw the woman's identification with her mother as an important determinant of her attitude toward motherhood and of her mothering behavior, the central role of the identification with the mother in the *wish* for motherhood was not particularly emphasized. They searched for explanations of this wish in biological or instinctual origins of mothering behavior. Adult women's psychological attitudes toward pregnancy and children were thought to some degree to be dependent on a hormonal or other biological basis, at least.

In recent years, we have witnessed a return to ideas expressed earlier by Horney (1926) and Thompson (1950), namely that childbearing has its origin in positive feminine identity and in identification with the reproductive function of the mother, rather than being substitutive or reparative (Tyson 1982) or resting entirely on a biological basis.

The role of the infant in eliciting responses from the caretaker is now thought to be important in the development of motherly feelings. Maternal feelings are understood as a response to the infant's needs and to the experience of caring for the baby (Klaus and Kennell 1976; Stern 1974). The concepts of attachment elaborated by Bowlby (1969) and Spitz and Wolf (1946) to describe the process of the development of a strong relationship between the infant and parent have been extended to include the development of the parent's attachment also (Ainsworth 1973; Brazelton et al. 1974; Kennell and Klaus 1983).

Femininity

To understand reproductive psychology (pregnancy) and pregnancy more broadly, we need to reconsider ideas about femininity and feminine development. *Femininity* is a complex term with many different meanings. Descriptive and normative concepts about femininity have been confused with each other, and the role of culture and socialization in creating those characteristics and behaviors that were once thought to be innate, or intrinsically derived from sexual or reproductive roles, has been recognized. It is now accepted that early attitudes and the expectations of parents and caretakers that are evoked at the time the gender of the infant is determined specifically affect the behavior of the parents toward the baby (Moss 1967). In turn, these environmental influences interact with the infant's genetic potential to determine development, including the particular forms of expression of gender.

Many authors have considered feminine identity, and have attempted to develop a concept of femininity that is consistent with observations and research data, all based on standards of female rather than male development. This task remains incomplete and is complicated since the components of femininity are not uniformly agreed on. Sociocultural variables are extremely important in all concepts of normality, including femininity (Clower 1976; Kleeman 1976; Parens et al. 1976; Stoller 1964, 1968, 1976; Tyson 1982).

Erikson (1964) proposed a concept of feminine identity formation that was not based on the "missing penis" but on what *was* part of the female body. He stated that "the female child . . . is disposed to observe evidence in older girls and women and in female animals of the fact that an inner-bodily space with productive as well as dangerous potentials does exist" (p. 267). He presented observations of the play of preadolescent children aged 10, 11, and 12 years to document the differences between "male and female spaces." Although he recognized the contribution of societal influences in the thinking and behavior of children of that age who have by then already developed clear gender role concepts, he at first believed these "male and female spaces" represented the awareness of fundamental differences related to the differences in "the groundplan of the human body." Erikson described the "critical importance of women's procreative task" as a way of being "uniquely creative" at the same time that he emphasized the new potential for intellectual, communal, and political participation of women.

Although this view of feminine identity formation based on a "female space" represents a recognition of the positive source of femininity, it has been criticized for ignoring the importance of early stereotyping socialization. However, Erikson did present a description of feminine development that considered the symbolic representations of the female body and its potential for pregnancy.

Some new concepts have emerged. Stoller (1976) differentiated the term *sex* as referring to biological character, including genetic endowment, genitals, and hormonal functioning, from *gender*, which is defined as the psychological and cultural concomitants of sex. *Core gender identity* is defined as the child's perception of himself or herself as a boy or girl. This perception begins to form as soon as the girl's parents recognize her as female.

Stoller's concept of "primary femininity" (1976) refers to a femininity derived from the early relationship with the mother. Body ego and self-identity derive from the girl's identification with someone whose body is the same as hers. Bodily sensations become part of the self-concept and are connected with "knowing" that one's own body can eventually bear children, as the mother's body can. The second, post-oedipal phase in the development of femininity results from resolution of the oedipal conflict and contributes another layer of femininity (Stoller 1976). These concepts describe the development of girls not as a variant of boys (i.e., as missing something and being defective), but following a separate line of growth. Tyson (1982) described a "developmental line of gender-identity, gender role, and choice of love object" (p. 74). The discovery of the anatomic difference between the sexes is understood as contributing to the development of symbolic thinking and to the capacity for wishful fantasy.

The wish for a baby is part of this development. It has been reported early (Parens et al. 1976) and can be understood as a manifestation of gender-role identification and feminine and maternal ego-ideal (Blum 1976). Menarche and adolescence provide stimuli for the further development of gender identity. New relationships in adolescence can alter concepts of femininity, including expectations of childbearing.

Psychological Preparedness for Pregnancy

Pregnancy demands the capacity to adapt to the "invasion" of one's body, to nurture the "parasite" as part of oneself, and also regard the developing baby as a separate being. It is first part of the mother and then increasingly a creature with a life and form of its own. Tolerance of this benign intrusion and the growth of the baby within requires adaptation to changing internal boundaries between the self and others, as well as changes in body image.

The psychology literature on gender differences yields some findings that have been the subject of considerable discussion and that are interesting in this regard and may be meaningful in understanding this process. The women and men have different patterns of attachments (Gilligan 1982; Notman et al. 1986). In the process of maturation, attachments are not relinquished in girls to the extent that is considered normal in boys. In early childhood, maturation, separation, and individuation are achievements considered necessary to accomplish to develop into adulthood. The separation process does not necessarily imply aloneness, but the capacity to be an individual. The girl can move more readily between her more adult personality consolidating and her more childish attachments to parents (Blos 1980) than the boy and has more ready access to feelings about her early relationships and her dependent feelings. This flexibility about boundaries and attachments to objects is important for the capacity to tolerate a pregnancy and the ambiguity of the fetus and its boundaries.

Pregnancy as a Developmental Crisis

In the 1950s and 1960s, a number of longitudinal studies of pregnancy were conducted (Bibring et al. 1961; Wenner et al. 1969). The concepts presented were of pregnancy as a developmental experience or a "normal developmental crisis"; that means that a pregnancy presents the opportunity for a critical maturational experience. The concept of developmental crisis does not mean a crisis in the sense of an emergency.

Conflicts from earlier developmental periods can be revived during a pregnancy, requiring new and different resolutions. Menarche, pregnancy, and menopause can be thought to be significant turning points in the life of a woman: after each one, the woman is no longer the same as before. Bibring et al. (1959, 1961) defined the developmental process of pregnancy in terms of the woman's relationship with her sexual partner, herself, and the child.

The idea that pregnancy has a developmental function was introduced and developed by Benedek, and implied by others (Bibring et al. 1959, 1961; Deutsch 1945). This process involved the idea that the woman can regress during this time, with loosening of defenses and the potential for a new reorganization of these defenses and changes in her self-concept. Bibring et al. (1961) and Wenner et al. (1969) observed that pregnancy redefined femininity. The women in their studies were flooded with memories and feelings about their mothers. They described a struggle during pregnancy between identification and differentiation, and stressed the importance of the capacity for and tolerance of some of these feelings—that the pregnant woman is more in touch with them than she may be at other times. The importance of the relationship with the mother of early life was also confirmed (Wenner et al. 1969).

The Clinical Course of Pregnancy

The following is a brief overview of pregnancy and some factors relating to potential pathology. At the beginning, a woman is characteristically reacting to the news of the pregnancy and anticipated changes because of it. A first pregnancy is clearly the most significant in the transition to motherhood, but later pregnancies also evoke unresolved issues from earlier pregnancies or early experiences. Who this baby appears to be and where it fits in the sibling order, its sex, and the mother's life circumstances also are important in the significance of a particular pregnancy. Ambivalence about a pregnancy has not always been recognized as normal and probably universal in our culture. Even if the baby is wanted, the pregnancy is planned, and the circumstances are right, the demands for adaptation as well as the feelings evoked make most women have mixed feelings at times, or even resentment or hostility about the pregnancy. The fetus is, after all, a "foreign body" as well as part of the mother and the father. Some women enjoy their pregnancies but have difficulty relating to the baby. The pregnancy can be gratifying as a well-done performance of their bodies, narcissistically rewarding. The demands of the new human being who is the baby is another thing entirely. Extreme ambivalence or hostility is a sign of potential difficulty. Sometimes this has its origin in a difficult ambivalent relationship to the woman's mother. It becomes difficult for her to make the transition to being a mother herself, when her feelings about *her* mother are conflicted.

Sometimes symptoms appear at this time. Obsessional thoughts, disturbing dreams, and anxiety reactions can accompany a pregnancy in a person who was not symptomatic previously. Many of these respond to brief interventions aimed at offering an opportunity to express ambivalence, permission to be resentful, and support. Emotional lability, with rapid mood swings and unexpected reactivity to inner and outer experiences, sometimes is a surprise to the woman herself, and to her husband and family.

One of the central aspects of pregnancy is the emotional revival of the relationship to the mother in the form of emerging memories, fantasies, wishes, or feelings. The woman can feel nostalgia for her childhood or her mother. This is poignantly illustrated by a vignette of a young pregnant teenager who had been adopted as a child. When her adoptive family learned she was pregnant, she was criticized and rejected by her adoptive mother.

She was in a home for unwed mothers and was very depressed. She expressed her longing directly, saying: "When you have a baby growing inside of you, you want to be close to the person inside of who you grew." The relationship of the woman with her mother is important in determining how the pregnancy will go, particularly the first pregnancy, which turns the woman into a mother herself.

In the first trimester, the pregnant woman is also confronted with her own physical vulnerability, sometimes for the first time. Concerns about control and oral and other conflicts can be revived, stimulated by the need to restrict diet, alcohol, or medications. She can also feel enormously pleased at the success of becoming pregnant, with heightened self-esteem, feelings of "femininity," and closeness to other women. This can alternate with anxiety, depression, and ambivalence. It is important to remember that the wish for a baby and the preparation for motherhood are not the same as the responses to the actual pregnancy. The psychological work of the pregnancy consists of the emotional adaptation to having a growing organism inside of oneself that will become an independent person but also has to be treated and tolerated as part of oneself.

Quickening, or feeling life, usually occurs in the early part of the second trimester. Since it is a subjective sensation appearing before fetal movements are visible, it generally is described earlier by multiparas who are more familiar with their feelings. Since the availability of ultrasound and amplification of fetal heart sounds, the first indication of the fetus as a separate and complete creature is no longer dependent on quickening. Many women, and men, regard the ultrasound image as their first picture of the baby. The technologic advances have permitted fathers to have an earlier sense of the baby and an earlier relationship to it.

Amniocentesis can be reassuring and also disturbing. It is invasive and can be frightening. Women vary as to whether they welcome "high tech" monitoring of pregnancy and delivery or find it distressing and intrusive. The pregnancy becomes visible to the outside world as the uterus expands and rises above the symphysis pubis. This "showing" can be gratifying, fulfilling exhibitionistic wishes, and also embarrassing. The pregnancy is clear evidence of sexuality and may also constitute an announcement about sexual wishes associated with some guilt. The increase in size can also have the meaning of fulfillment of phallic fantasies as the body expands and protrudes. Growth of the breast size is also gratifying to women who felt their breasts to be inadequate. The second trimester is usually a time of relative well-being physically, accompanied by an increase in energy as compared to the first.

In the third trimester, the growth of the fetus to the point of distortion of the body can produce discomfort and is usually distressing to some degree. Thoughts of approaching labor and delivery can be preoccupying. Anxieties reflecting early childhood fantasies about impregnation and birth may be stirred up and can be focused on the delivery. Fantasies or concerns about the adequacy of the birth canal and about being damaged are common. Concerns about fetal abnormalities can reflect unconscious fantasies and guilt. If a woman feels inadequate or guilty, she may feel that someone as "imperfect" as she or as "bad" cannot possibly produce a "perfect" child. The tendency for the woman to take responsibility for whatever the outcome of the pregnancy ignores the role of the father and his genetic contribution. It does, however, reflect the traditional orientation of mothers who feel that the baby growing inside is intimately connected with them and determined by their good or bad selves and behavior. To some extent this is obviously true, since the placenta nourishes the baby and the mother's behavior affects the prenatal environment. But the importance of the tendency for women to take responsibility for whatever happens with children, realistic, nutritional, or not, is culturally strongly reinforced. The particular configuration of anxieties will be different for each woman according to her own orientation: for example, the expectation of suffering during delivery can be due to her mother's experience as well as to culturally influenced expectations.

During labor and delivery there is considerable variation in the extent to which a woman receives support. With the advent of sterile obstetrical technique, making it possible to prevent infection, the interpersonal as well as the surgical environment became sterile, and many young women who were living far from their extended family felt quite isolated, especially when fathers were not allowed in the delivery room. This has changed again in recent years. Currently, technologic methods (e.g., fetal monitoring) are widely used, and malpractice concerns can override emotional ones. Support in the process of labor and delivery is very important.

Pregnancy at Specific Developmental Stages

Pregnancy has most often been discussed as an experience for the mother or the family without specifically considering their actual life stage or life circumstances. A pregnancy in a teenager has a different impact than one for a woman in her mid-20s who has already separated from her family or for a woman in her mid-30s who has established a career. It is also different than for a woman who is approaching the end of her reproductive period. Her achievements, social environment supports available, and her own state of maturity can be quite varied. The potential of the pregnancy as a stimulus for maturation and for exploring her relationship to her mother and her capacity to relate to the baby and to its father will have been affected by her previous life experience.

An adolescent pregnancy and a pregnancy in a 40-year-old woman provide two models of different life phases. The adolescent simultaneously has to integrate development from childhood into being an adult woman and to adapt to the pregnancy itself. For most older women, pregnant for the first time, considerably more maturation has already occurred, with consolidation of their gender identity and greater personal development and individuation. Pre-oedipal aspects of her relationship with her mother have ordinarily been experienced in a number of ways in her life; choices have been made that have realized some of her potential capabilities and have sealed off others. She has formed relationships that bring into fruition some of her wishes, past fantasies, and talents.

The confirmation of femininity and of the healthy functioning of her body that a pregnancy makes possible has an additional dimension for the older woman. It can be particularly reassuring to her to feel that she is functioning properly, and that signs of aging that she may have perceived have not interfered with her reproductive responsibilities. The pregnancy can also stir up age-appropriate concerns. The growth of the uterus and the body expansion and distortion can give rise to uncertainties about her body and its normality. This can be displaced to anxiety about the fetus.

It is impressive that even in older primiparas whose lives are well established and who are well developed as individuals, a pregnancy can evoke strong feelings and unresolved aspects about the relationship with their mother. Some things remain quite similar: the opportunity for growth, unconscious guilt, fantasies and concern about damage, concern about dependence and independence, and concern about the capacity for caring and mothering.

A pregnancy can thus open a pathway for further exploration of feminine identification and present the possibility of new access to unconscious conflicts, wishes, and fantasies. It also ushers in a new phase of life with its potential for expanding feelings of belonging to the parental generation.

Currently, with the advent of new reproductive technology, women's strong wishes for having a baby biologically their own can be realized in situations that previously meant pregnancy was impossible. For some women, this has meant enormously important fulfillment. But the emotional and financial costs are high, and, for some, the dilemmas as to how far to proceed, when to persist, and when to stop have been difficult.

Discovering ways to achieve the development and gratifications of a pregnancy can be helped by a fuller understanding of pregnancy itself.

References

Ainsworth M: The development of infant-mother attachments, in Review of Child Development Research, Vol 3. Edited by Caldwell BM, Ricciuti HN. Chicago, IL, University of Chicago Press, 1973

Benedek T: Parenthood as a developmental phase. J Am Psychoanal Assoc 7:379–417, 1959

Benedek T: The psychobiology of pregnancy, in Parenthood: Its Psychology and

Psychopathology. Edited by Anthony EJ, Benedek T. Boston, MA, Little, Brown, 1970, pp 137–151

Benedek T, Rubenstein B: Psychosexual Functions in Women. New York, Rouard Press, 1952

Bibring G: Some considerations of the psychological processes in pregnancy. Psychoanal Study Child 14:113–121, 1959

Bibring G, Dwyer TF, Huntington DS, et al: A study of the psychological processes in pregnancy and of the earliest mother-child relationship. Psychoanal Study Child 16:9–72, 1961

Blos P: Modification in the traditional psychoanalytic theory of juvenile adolescents' development. Adolesc Psychiatry 8:8–24, 1980

Blum H: Masochism, the ego ideal, and the psychology of women. J Am Psychoanal Assoc 24:157–191, 1976

Bowlby J: Attachment and loss, Vol 1: Attachment. London, Hogarth Press, 1969

Brazelton TB, Koslowski B, Main M: The origins of reciprocity: the early mother-infant interaction, in The Effect of the Infant on Its Caregiver. Edited by Lewis M, Rosenblum L. New York, John Wiley, 1974

Chasseguet-Smirgel J: Feminine guilt and the oedipus couple (1970), in Female Sexuality. Edited by Chasseguet-Smirgel J. Ann Arbor, MI, University of Michigan Press, 1970, pp 94–134

Clower V: Theoretical implications of current views of masturbation in latency girls. J Am Psychoanal Assoc 24 (suppl):109–125, 1976

Deutsch H: The Psychology of Women, Vol 1. New York, Grune & Stratton, 1944

Deutsch H: The Psychology of Women, Vol 2. New York, Grune & Stratton, 1945

Erikson EH: Childhood and Society, 2nd Edition. New York, WW Norton, 1963

Erikson E: Inner and outer space: reflections on womanhood. Daedalus 93:582–608, 1964

Freud S: Three essays on the theory of sexuality (1905), in The Standard Edition of the Complete Psychological Works of Sigmund Freud, Vol 7. Translated and edited by Strachey J. London, Hogarth Press, 1962, pp 261–285

Freud S: Some psychical consequences of the anatomical distinction between the sexes (1925), in The Standard Edition of the Complete Psychological Works of Sigmund Freud, Vol 19. Translated and edited by Strachey J. London, Hogarth Press, 1962, pp 248–258

Freud S: Femininity (1932), in The Standard Edition of the Complete Psychological Works of Sigmund Freud, Vol 22. Translated and edited by Strachey J. London, Hogarth Press, 1962, pp 112–135

Gilligan C: In a Different Voice. Cambridge, MA, Harvard University Press, 1982

Horney K: The flight from womanhood. Int J Psychoanal 7:324–339, 1926

Kennell JH, Klaus MH: Early events: later effects on the infant, in Frontiers of Infant Psychiatry. Edited by Cale J, Galenson E, Tyson R. New York, Basic Books, 1983

Kestenberg J: Regression and reintegration in pregnancy. J Am Psychoanal Assoc 24:213–250, 1976

Klaus M, Kennell J: Maternal Infant Bonding: The Impact of Early Separation or Loss on Family Development. St. Louis, MO, CV Mosby, 1976

Kleeman JA: Freud's views on early female sexuality in the light of direct child observation. J Am Psychoanal Assoc 24:3–27, 1976

Moss HA: Sex, age and state as determinants of mother-infant interaction. Merril-Palmer Quarterly 13:19–36, 1967

Notman MT, Zilbach JJ, Baker-Miller J, et al: Themes in psychoanalytic understanding of women: some reconsiderations of autonomy and affiliation. J Am Acad Psychoanal 14:241–253, 1986

Parens H (reporter): Parenthood as a developmental phase (panel). J Am Psychoanal Assoc 23:154–165, 1975

Parens H, Pollock L, Stein J, et al: On the girl's entry into the Oedipus complex. J Am Psychoanal Assoc 24:79–107, 1976

Sadow L: The psychological origins of parenthood, in Parent hood. Edited by Cohen RS, Cohler BJ, Weissman SH. New York, Guilford, 1984, pp 285–296

Schwartz D: Psychoanalytic developmental perspectives on parenthood, in Parenthood. Edited by Cohen RS, Cohler BJ, Weissman SH. New York, Guilford, 1984, pp 356–372

Spitz R, Wolf K: The smiling response: a contribution to the ontogenesis of social relations. Genetic Psychology Monographs 34:57–125, 1946

Stern D: Mother and infant at play: the dyadic interaction involving facial, vocal and gaze behavior, in The Effect of the Infant on Its Caregiver. Edited by Lewis M, Rosenblum L. New York, John Wiley, 1974, pp 187–215

Stoller R: A contribution to the study of gender identity. Int J Psychoanal 45:220–226, 1964

Stoller R: The sense of femaleness. Psychoanal Q 37:42–55, 1968

Stoller R: Primary femininity. J Am Psychoanal Assoc 24:59–78, 1976

Thompson C: Some effects of the derogatory attitude towards female sexuality. Psychiatry 13:349–354, 1950

Tyson P: A developmental line of gender identity, gender role, and choice of love object. J Am Psychoanal Assoc 30:61–86, 1982

Wenner NK, Cohen MB, Weigert EV, et al: Emotional problems in pregnancy. Psychiatry 32:389–410, 1969

Chapter 3

Male Gender-Related Issues in Reproduction and Technology

Michael F. Myers, M.D., F.R.C.P.(C)

It is estimated that 15–20% of married couples have an infertility problem (Kraft et al. 1980); that is, they have been unable to achieve a successful pregnancy after a year of regular sexual relations without contraception (Mazor 1978). As more couples are postponing childbearing until they are in their 30s or 40s, this estimate may increase. This means that significant numbers of individuals who undergo infertility studies and who approach infertility experts for reproductive counseling and technological assistance are reacting psychologically to the frustration of not being able to conceive with ease. How do men react to, and cope with, infertility?

Mourning of one's anticipated, or assumed, ability to have a child always accompanies the threat of or the reality of infertility. Although one is never completely certain of being fertile until it is proven, many individuals, especially individuals who have enjoyed good health, take their reproductive capacity for granted. When it becomes increasingly evident that fertility is either difficult, delayed, or impossible, most individuals begin to mourn (Spencer 1987). All stages of bereavement are common—denial, shock, anger, bargaining, depression, and acceptance—and men vary enormously on how they progress through the various stages of mourning.

I am grateful to Drs. Christo Zouves, Peter McComb, Gerald Korn, and Andrew Moore for their time and helpful suggestions regarding the in vitro fertilization, artificial insemination by donor, and vasovasostomy portions of this chapter.

Because men are less expressive and do not talk about their feelings as readily or as openly as women, their distress may be missed. Further, many husbands feel the need to be strong, steady, and available for their wives. This is an adaptive and sex-role–related response that many couples employ to preserve their marital integrity and solidarity while trying to become pregnant. It is unusual to see the roles reversed, where the husband is quite symptomatic and particularly down at each menstrual period, and his wife is cool and in control. Sometimes, both the husband and wife are demoralized, sad, and bitter, but again not often at the same time. Occasionally, the husband's self-control and calmness are misconstrued by his wife as lack of interest and lack of feeling, which can become a problem if they are not able to communicate easily with each other.

When it is the man himself who is infertile, he may have a characteristic "cast" to his mourning. He may become reflective, brooding, and withdrawn. His wife may have difficulty getting him to talk about his feelings, and he may reject her outright. He may obsess about being defective, inadequate, or less of a man (Mahlstedt 1985), and if he (or his family) has a history of depression, he may become clinically depressed. His gender identity (i.e., his inner sense of maleness and masculinity) may become affected as he derides himself for "shooting blanks," the common colloquialism for azoospermia, if that is the reason for the infertility. Some men lose interest in sex with their wives, and they may develop psychogenic impotence. This may lead to even more pulling away and withdrawal with enhanced isolation, shame, and guilty ruminations. Needless to say, couples who have problems with infertility have marriages that are more stressed (Pohlman 1970).

There are strong sociocultural expectancies in favor of procreation and parenthood. This holds for both women and men. One need listen only to couples who are childless by choice to receive an education in social stigmatization; these individuals describe being subject to intense pressure from their families, friends, and co-workers to have children, and they are made to feel deviant for not wanting children. These societal values, plus religious customs and beliefs, become incorporated into a man's thinking and outlook about fatherhood. In at least one religion, Judaism, fatherhood is central to the man's understanding of his obligations to his community and to God (Gold 1988). In ancient Jewish law, a man who is not a father is incomplete.

My clinical impression is that more men than women have a high need for secrecy and privacy regarding their infertility. This holds whether the infertility problem rests with themselves, their wives, or them both. This sense of not wanting to discuss "their problem" with others is often part of the general sense of privacy that most husbands have about marital matters. In some marriages, husbands are very controlling about this issue; their wives feel inhibited, restrained, and eventually resentful that they are not "allowed" to talk to anyone. Infertile couples already feel a sense of isolation and alienation from others, in that they are grieving, and there are no formal rituals or supports (Mazor 1978). This isolation is magnified for the woman who must keep her feelings to herself to protect her husband's wishes.

Diagnostic Investigations and Treatment Programs

How do men react to infertility investigations and treatments? First, at no other time in their lives have most men felt so exposed. Not only are they subjected to a series of medical questions, a physical examination, and laboratory tests, but they are asked the most personal questions about their psychological functioning, their marital lives, and their sexuality. If these men are not accustomed to talking frankly about themselves to health care professionals, and if the latter are not particularly experienced or sensitive to delicate matters when working with men of infertile couples, the entire diagnostic and investigative process can become quite an ordeal. The man may develop a feeling of being assaulted, that there has been an invasion of his body, his feelings, his inner self. This feeling may be even more pronounced if he has no information whatsoever about what to expect and has not done any reading to prepare himself.

Some men have a lot of feelings about semen collection and analysis. Not only might they be anxious about the results but they are often anxious about masturbating on demand to provide a specimen. If they are timid, awkward, or inhibited they will feel self-conscious about giving a specimen in the clinic, "in the bathroom down the hall." They may feel that they are performing a very private act (and an act that some men, especially Roman Catholic men, have ambivalent feelings about) in a public setting. Carrying semen around in a jar may make them anxious and embarrassed. They may have regressive fantasies of feeling naked, exposed, or "dirty." These are not feelings that men talk easily about; they are more likely to hide them behind a joking demeanor or a posture of bravado.

Attempting to become pregnant by scheduling intercourse at the time of ovulation each month can become difficult after awhile, no matter how much couples try to relax, try to be versatile, or try to use humor. Many husbands begin to feel the pressure of intercourse on demand; they feel objectified, that they are a machine that deposits sperm once a month. Sexual intercourse becomes a chore, or work, and is no longer erotically pleasurable for either the husband or his wife. Once he ejaculates, he has done his "job," and his wife no longer wants or needs him—until the next time. Each month becomes a bit of an emotional roller coaster as his hopes soar, only to be dashed when his wife's menstrual period begins.

Here is what one man has to say about his experience with infertility: "It's strange that when you're trying to create life, death is so often on your mind. Every time my wife got her period, it was like a small touch of death. A funeral for what never existed" (Jacobson 1987, p. 50).

Many women express a need to talk about their range of feelings in response to infertility fears and to the infertility investigation itself. In this way, they feel a bit better, more energized to persevere, and more connected to their husbands. Unfortunately, many husbands feel just the opposite (Valentine 1986). They argue that talking about the procedures and the doctors' visits makes them feel worse. They too find the whole process tedious, exhausting, and discouraging but they try to deal with it differently by not thinking about it. Further, as long as they retain a sense of medical hope (Snarey et al. 1986) of having a child in the future, they are more likely to remain patient about having this child, as opposed to considering adoption or child-free living.

Reactions to In Vitro Fertilization

Most men who present with their wives for in vitro fertilization (IVF) are still struggling with psychological sequelae to their infertility. In one study, 15% of the men reported that infertility was the most upsetting experience of their lives (Freeman et al. 1985). In another study, 26% of the men had symptoms of a mood disorder at the beginning of IVF and an exacerbation of these symptoms after an unsuccessful attempt at IVF (Garner et al. 1984). Assessing the sexual functioning and psychological status of 45 married couples requesting IVF, Fagan et al. (1986) noted that 10 of the men had either a sexual dysfunction or a psychiatric disorder, using DSM-III (American Psychiatric Association 1980) criteria. By way of contrast, in their study of 300 couples admitted to an IVF program, Hearn et al. (1987) found that their subjects reported good quality of life and freedom from anxiety and depression.

The earlier and more completely that men are included in the IVF examination and counseling, the better. Not only does this involve them as active participants, which they are, it also will decrease any sense of isolation, self-imposed or otherwise, that they may feel. Husbands are not as likely then to develop irrational fantasies about their marital and sexual lives being exposed by their wives to the IVF doctors without their consent. When the obstetrician is male, and the husband has been involved from the beginning of treatment, there is less danger that the man will worry about the doctor touching and examining his wife. He will also have fewer competitive feelings with the male physician because he knows and trusts him. When the husband is also allowed to be present in the examining room (with his wife's consent), his knowledge about reproductive physiology, gynecologic examinations, and the IVF procedures is enhanced.

There have been reports in both the lay press (Landsberg 1987a, 1987b; Lasker and Borg 1987) and the medical literature (Black et al. 1987; Nordlicht 1987) about exploitation of the infertile couple. I won't go into the myriad ethical matters that arise from the new reproductive technologies because they are covered elsewhere (Lantos, Chapter 7, this volume). However, the more honestly informed the husband is about the IVF procedure itself, and the clinic's advertised success rate, the better he will be able to cooperate with the program and not feel angry or misled. The bottom line is that infertile couples are really interested in knowing the percentage of IVF couples in their age-group with their particular problem who take home a baby. They do not want figures that are inflated and are based on pregnancy rates in general.

Here are some issues that have proven to be clinically significant and fairly common. In working with couples in which the woman is obviously better informed about the technical aspects of IVF than the man, it is important to try to understand why. Has he not done as much reading or talked to other people with infertility problems as she has? Is he as interested in proceeding with IVF or is he just being swept along in some ways? Does he fully understand his part in the procedure and does he have any questions? Does he have concerns about getting away from work to be at the clinic when required? Is he worried about the invasive procedures his wife must undergo and the drugs she must take? Does he have unrealistic, science-fiction fantasies about "test-tube babies"? Does he have mixed feelings about the possibility of having multiple births if the IVF is successful? Does he have religious or moral conflicts about the scientific and mechanical nature of conception, as opposed to "natural conception through an act of love"? These are important questions that husbands must be encouraged to talk about during the assessment and counseling period.

With regard to the decision to embrace IVF in the first place, how much does male "control" in the marital relationship play a part? Lorber (1988) argued that despite our culture's emphasis on motherhood, the man is often the dominant partner in reproductive decisions. She cited the work of Crowe (1985), who concluded that IVF is not value-neutral and who found a certain degree of ambivalence toward IVF in her study of Australian women who had had IVF treatment. Lorber also referred to the increasing popularity of IVF in cases of male infertility, especially low sperm count (oligospermia), low sperm motility (asthenospermia), and abnormal sperm morphology (teratospermia). However, gender politics—that is, women are socialized to give, to serve others, and to be subordinates (Miller 1976)—may be at work here because of men's strong investment in biological parenthood and women's willingness to take on the physiologic responsibility for treatment. The failure to fertilize a "good egg" is a male problem; the failure of a successfully fertilized embryo to implant in the womb is more likely to be perceived as a female problem.

Artificial Insemination by Donor Programs

Thousands of babies are conceived each year by artificial insemination by donor, and this technology has offered hope to many infertile couples. The decision to have artificial insemination is not an easy one for the couple to reach, and it is especially difficult for the man. Notman (1984) stated that it is not unusual for husbands to have many feelings at the same time. In one way, an unequal situation is created by the woman's having the intimate experience of pregnancy; her husband is not a biological part of her pregnancy. However, husbands can be very positive and supportive of their wives' joy in being pregnant, while simultaneously having doubts about pregnancy resulting from artificial insemination by a donor. Husbands worry about the pregnancy itself, then the baby's appearance, and whether there will be any resemblance to them. Husbands also have concerns of a legal nature regarding the biological father's rights as opposed to their own. Husbands feel very private about the decision to use artificial insemination, which will not be a problem if their wives feel the same way. Men who are raised as Catholics but who are no longer practicing, or who have converted to another faith, may retain moral conflicts about artificial insemination by donor. They feel guilty, or that they have sinned, and that artificial insemination by donor is an adulterous act to which they are an accomplice. More recently, since acquired immunodeficiency syndrome (AIDS) has become a worry, some men fear that the donors themselves might be positive for the human immunodeficiency virus (HIV) antibody.

Berger et al. (1986) recommended that couples should wait at least 3 months between discovery of an infertility problem and embarking on an artificial insemination by donor program. This gives each of the individuals, but especially the husband, an opportunity to begin to adapt to the infertility when the problem resides with him. These same authors have also noted in their work with couples that many have mixed feelings about secrecy. They found that husbands whose wives had not yet conceived by artificial insemination by donor were more willing to discuss their infertility with others than were husbands whose wives had already conceived. They postulate that applicants of an artificial insemination by donor program find discussing their infertility concerns and the procedure psychologically helpful; secrecy once they conceive is perhaps one measure of their sense of relief. It may also represent denial of a fertility problem and a need to bond in an adaptive sense with the developing fetus.

Unconscious factors for infertile husbands embarking on an artificial insemination by donor program must not be dismissed. Such issues as feelings of competition with the donor, envy of the donor, or hostile rivalry toward the donor may surface in dreams or later in displaced form in their everyday relationships with men. Infertile husbands who retain feelings of inferiority or incompleteness, plus anger at being infertile in the first place, may have difficulty getting along with other men because of their defensive abrasiveness toward others. Other men may be isolative and not have any male friends. If their relationships with men were already a problem because of the particular psychosocial dynamics of their growing-up years, then they may be even worse on discovering their infertility and embarking on an artificial insemination by donor program. Fortunately for most husbands, once the baby is born and a relationship begins between the child and his or her father, the majority of concerns and anxieties fade away.

One can only speculate about whether or not there is actual emotional distancing by the husband during the entire undertaking, and perhaps during the pregnancy also, to some degree, until the baby is born. Husbands do have questions about the physical characteristics of the donors, and quite understandably so. Despite explanation and reassurance from the doctors about matching the physical and ethnic traits of the donors as closely as possible with those of the husbands, it may be possible that many men cannot really relax about the whole experience until they actually see their baby. At that point, their worst fears are laid to rest.

Sperm Donors

The two most common reasons why men become sperm donors are humanitarian and financial (G. Korn, personal communication). Most donors are single young men or monogamous married men with some college education; many are undergraduates and many are postgraduate students. A comprehensive family and personal history is obtained to screen for inheritable diseases. Homosexual and bisexual men are not accepted. The American Fertility Society recommends blood testing for venereal disease, cytomegalovirus, hepatitis B, and AIDS. At present, AIDS testing is done every 6 months on donors, and, because of delayed seroconversion in people who are exposed to the AIDS virus, most clinics are now using only frozen sperm as a precautionary measure.

There are a number of ethical and legal issues for sperm donors and artificial insemination by donor programs to consider (Andrews 1987). When there is an informed consent form for the donor to sign, he will then know how his sperm is being used and how often. He will understand confidentiality guidelines and what information about him is being disclosed to the recipients of his sperm. But what if something turns up in his medical screening examination about which he is not aware? What becomes of the doctor's records? Can the donor's identity be traced in any manner? Could a donor be held financially liable as the biological father of a child he has never seen or raised? Some donors may feel fine about their sperm being used for inseminations at the discretion of the doctor or clinic. Others may not want their sperm used for single women, especially lesbian women.

There are two other matters for men who are sperm donors. Some men have reported feeling remorseful about donating sperm for the creation of children with whom they have no contact (Andrews 1985). This is a feeling that they have later when they have had children in a marriage and have a sense of being a father. Some men may not have a remorseful feeling but yet have a feeling of discomfort after awhile. One man described his feelings in this manner: "I was glad when it ended after a year. I was starting to feel uncomfortable about possibly having so many children that I don't know. The closer I came to starting my own family, the more real the idea of fathering became for me" (Lasker and Borg 1987, p. 106). Other men have reported concerns much later when their own children are grown; they fear the possibility of a consanguineous marriage occurring between one of the children of their marriage and one of the individuals who has been conceived from their sperm donation.

It is difficult to know how powerful the financial motive is for some donors. Students are notoriously hard pressed for money, and becoming a sperm donor is an easy way to make money. It is hoped, of course, that donors take the responsibility seriously and do not lie about, or unconsciously gloss over, their personal and family histories. Donors may not have the personal maturity to appreciate fully the emotional distress of childless couples. Occasionally a member of their family or a close personal friend is struggling with the problem. It is quite possible that, at least for some men, being a sperm donor fulfills a need to prove one's masculinity and sexual prowess as a man. Their motive may be narcissistic and self-serving, rather than humanitarian.

Technical Advances in Vasovasostomy (Vas Deferens Reanastomosis) Procedures

With large numbers of divorced men remarrying younger women, vasectomy reversal has become a commonly requested operation. Hence, any technical urologic advances in both vasectomy procedures and in their reversal are generally well received by men. Not only are these operations now more simple, the chances of the man's sperm count and sperm motility returning to an acceptable standard for vas deferens reanastomosis are now much better than they were a decade ago. The shorter the interval between vasectomy and vasectomy reversal, the better the outcome. After 10 years, the results are less positive (A.J. Moore, personal communication).

It has long been known that most men who are fathers, and who request a vasectomy, have thought long and hard about the permanence of the procedure. They have had as many children as they want, and they do not envision having children ever again. Most men do not like to think about one of their children dying (which might make them want to consider having another child later) or their marriage, perceived to be stable, ending. Even after divorce, many men who have had vasectomies remain clear that they do not wish to have more children in a new or future relationship. When they are certain of this and communicate their feelings unambivalently to their partner, this enables the woman to decide very early whether to pursue the relationship or not. Other men, however, find that their feelings about having more children do change in the context of a happy, loving, and exciting relationship with someone new. This is especially likely to happen to those men who were unhappily married for a long period of time and whose memories of family life are unpleasant because of so much tension or fighting or coldness at home.

But there are other dynamics for men who are anxious to have more children and who are grateful that their fertility may possibly be restored. Some of these men married at a very young age the first time around. They had children when they were immature and knew very little about being a father. Many report that they missed out on many nurturant and interactive aspects of their children's lives because they were working so hard (or "playing" so hard with their male friends) and were rarely at home. These men, now in their late 30s or early 40s, have children who are grown and to whom they may not feel gratifyingly close. For them to have another chance, to start again and to be a more involved father is challenging and stimulating.

Other divorced men in new relationships may be struggling with aging and issues of mid-life. To be with a younger woman, and to be starting a family, is invigorating and, for them, restorative of their youth. They feel younger and act younger (Myers 1989). Many describe this phase of their life as a second life, or a new life; their attitude and approach to this marriage and starting a family is very different than before. These men have much more financial security as they embark on this "new life" than they did in their earlier marriage.

Some divorced men may be working out an intrapsychic conflict by having their vasectomy reversed and their fertility restored. This conflict may be related to the damage to their self-esteem, usefulness, and masculinity as a consequence of the divorce. I have seen this from time to time in divorced men who were totally against the divorce and who felt completely aban-doned by their wives (Myers 1985). This narcissistic injury cuts to their very core: by having their fertility back, they feel more whole. They then view themselves as more worthy, more desirable, and more lovable as they begin to reenter the "singles" world and try to form a new and significant lasting relationship. This was signified by one man who reported to me after his vasectomy reversal: "I don't feel like damaged goods anymore." He felt he could now compete "with the best of them." Other men begin to talk about having their vasectomies reversed while they are still with their wives but have not yet separated. They have reached the point in their marriages where divorce has now become inevitable. These men are already projecting into the future and beginning to plan their lives vis-à-vis new relationships.

Conclusion

In this chapter, I have attempted to address some of the issues for men regarding the new reproductive technologies. This is merely a beginning as there are few data about men who are the patients and men who are the doctors in this branch of clinical medicine. There is danger in equating men's silence about reproduction with acceptance and cooperation. We must ask more questions and chip away at the wall of silence. Only in this way can we increase our knowledge base and refine our diagnostic and treatment approaches to women and men with reproductive problems.

References

American Psychiatric Association: Diagnostic and Statistical Manual of Mental Disorders, 3rd Edition. Washington, DC, American Psychiatric Association, 1980

Andrews LB: New Conceptions: A Consumers Guide to the Newest Fertility Treatments Including In Vitro Fertilization, Artificial Insemination, and Surrogate Motherhood. New York, Ballantine, 1985

Andrews LB: Ethical and legal aspects of in-vitro fertilization and artificial insemination by donor. Urol Clin North Am 14:633–642, 1987

Berger DM, Eisen A, Shuber J, et al: Psychological patterns in donor insemination couples. Can J Psychiatry 31:818–823, 1986

Blackwell RE, Carr BR, Chang RJ, et al: Are we exploiting the infertile couple? Fertil Steril 48:735–739, 1987

Crowe C: "Women want it": in vitro fertilization and women's motivations for participation. Women's Studies International Forum 8:57–62, 1985

Fagan PJ, Schmidt CW Jr, Rock JA, et al: Sexual functioning and psychologic evaluation of in vitro fertilization couples. Fertil Steril 46:668–672, 1986

Freeman EW, Boxer AS, Rickels K, et al: Psychological evaluation and support in a program of in vitro fertilization and embryo transfer. Fertil Steril 43:48–53, 1985

Garner CH, Arnold EW, Gray H: The psychological impact of in vitro fertilization (abstract). Fertil Steril 41:13S, 1984

Gold M: The real Jewish father, in A Mensch Among Men: Explorations in Jewish Masculinity. Edited by Brod H. Freedom, CA, Crossing Press, 1988, pp 84–91

Hearn MT, Yuzpe AA, Brown SE, et al: Psychological characteristics of in vitro fertilization participants. Am J Obstet Gynecol 156:269–274, 1987

Jacobson M: The baby chase. Esquire Magazine, May 1987, pp 49–50

Kraft AD, Polombo J, Mitchell D, et al: The psychological dimensions of infertility. Am J Orthopsychiatry 50:618–622, 1980

Landsberg M: Guinea pigs of test-tube fertilization have second thoughts. The Globe and Mail, August 15, 1987a

Landsberg M: Truth about in vitro fertilization overshadowed by the hype. The Globe and Mail, August 22, 1987b

Lasker JN, Borg S: In Search of Parenthood: Coping With Infertility and High-tech Conception. Boston, MA, Beacon, 1987

Lorber J: In vitro fertilization and gender politics, in Women and Health: Special Issue:

Embryos, Ethics, and Women's Rights: Exploring the New Reproductive Technologies. Edited by Baruch EH, D'Adamo AF Jr, Seager J. New York, Haworth, 1988, pp 117–133

Mahlstedt P: The psychological component of infertility. Fertil Steril 43:335–346, 1985

Mazor MD: The problem of infertility, in The Woman Patient: Medical and Psychological Interfaces, Vol 1: Sexual and Reproductive Aspects of Women's Health Care. Edited by Notman MT, Nadelson CC. New York, Plenum, 1978, pp 137–160

Miller JB: Toward a New Psychology of Women. Boston, MA, Beacon, 1976

Myers MF: Angry abandoned husbands: assessment and treatment, in Men's Changing Roles in the Family. Edited by Lewis RA, Sussman MB. New York, Haworth, 1985, pp 31–42

Myers MF: Men and Divorce. New York, Guilford, 1989

Nordlicht S: Humanism and medical ethics in a technological age. NY State J Med 87:427–428, 1987

Notman MT: Psychological aspects of AID, in Infertility: Medical, Emotional, and Social Considerations. Edited by Mazor MD, Simons HF. New York, Human Sciences Press, 1984, pp 145–153

Pohlman E: Childlessness, intentional and unintentional. J Nerv Ment Dis 151:2–12, 1970

Snarey J, Son L, Kuehne V: How husbands cope when pregnancy fails: a longitudinal study of infertility and psychosocial generativity (working paper). Wellesley, MA, Wellesley College Center for Research on Women, 1986

Spencer L: Male infertility: 5 psychological correlates. Postgrad Med 81:223–228, 1987

Valentine DP: Psychological impact of infertility: identifying issues and needs. Soc Work Health Care 11:61–69, 1986

Chapter 4

Lessons to Be Learned From the DES Experience

Roberta J. Apfel, M.D., M.P.H.
Susan M. Fisher, M.D.

Diethylstilbestrol (DES) is a synthetic estrogenic pill that was heralded with the same enthusiasm that has greeted other medical technologies. All elements of medical practice that are knowledge based—drugs, techniques, equipment, and procedures used by health care professionals—are subsumed under the general definition of technologies. All the newer reproductive technologies are similar to DES in that they represent hope and promise, they tend to be adopted into general use before they have been fully evaluated, and they continue to be used even after they have been shown to be unsafe or ineffective. The more recently introduced reproductive technologies bring with them the same wishes that led to the prescription of DES. The newer technologies are increasingly complex and have a power to create and to damage that is proportional to their complexity. There is always a tension between progress and caution. While we encourage and applaud progress, we also need to heed the DES story, which is a cautionary tale based on earlier progress.

The DES Story and Current Parallels

DES became popularized as a pregnancy treatment that could bring babies to women who were at high risk for losing pregnancies. The technique, called the "Smith and Smith Regime," was developed by a husband and wife team at the Fearing Research Laboratory at Harvard Medical School (Smith and Smith 1949). This laboratory is still functioning; now researchers study men as well as women, and they are beginning to explain how the immune and

37

reproductive systems interact at a molecular level. These exciting new vistas of human knowledge and understanding usher in new technologies by which science may alter the natural course of events. These alterations bring their own iatrogenic problems. The DES story is a cautionary tale about how unpredicted damage and risk, in retrospect, outweigh what seemed 50 years ago to be pure benefit. Furthermore, in the DES story, the damage and risk continue to unfold; reproductive cancer, infertility, and central nervous system effects of DES will be discussed in this chapter. The risk-benefit ratios are even higher today.

DES is one of many synthetic estrogenic hormone medications that evolved from the popular sex hormone treatments that became available in the 1920s. Estrogens were considered the source of female youthfulness and were introduced as therapies for everything from menopause to hives. Charles Dodds, the scientist who was knighted for his synthesis of DES in 1928, wrote in 1924: "It is difficult to call to mind any subject upon which more rubbish has been written than the sex hormones. This is very largely the result of the general public's desire for the maintenance of youth and all that it implies, together with the successful exploitation of this trait by commercial firms" (Dodds 1934). Even when natural estrogens could be administered only by injection and caused abscesses, they were popular; the inexpensive orally administered substitute DES was destined to become even more popular (Apfel and Fisher 1984).

The recent excitement over tretinoin (RETIN-A), a substance similarly touted as an answer to the scars and wrinkles of aging skin, is a similar reminder of that universal wish for youth (*The New York Times* 1988). DES was, moreover, a sex hormone, and thereby appealed to additional universal wishes for sexuality, potency, and fertility. DES was initially approved for a limited number of conditions by the U.S. Food and Drug Administration (FDA) in 1941, after an unprecedented amount of study and discussion. Once it was marketed, the indications for usage broadened. By 1947, the DES pill had been approved in a larger dosage for pregnancy use. The Smiths, who developed the DES prescription in pregnancy, believed that this estrogen would redress an imbalance in the hormones of the placenta of women who had previously miscarried and would enable them to carry their babies to term (Smith 1948).

Initially DES was used for "habitual aborters"—women who had spontaneously aborted more than one pregnancy and whose risk of abortion increased in subsequent pregnancies. Diabetic women who have difficulty carrying pregnancies to term were reported to have more successful pregnancies with DES. Then the treatment was expanded; it was even used for normal women in their first pregnancies. This is typical of the easy extension to a broader population base that frequently occurs when a promising new treatment comes along. Soon DES was being used "prophylactically" and "to make normal babies even more normal." It was included in prenatal vitamins ("Desplex"), in a hair tonic ("Stilbepan"), and in "sex pills" ("Prolific") (Direcks 1987). The drug was given for a range of reasons, some quite legitimate, which continue to this day (e.g., to suppress tumor growth in men with prostate cancer). Other uses for DES were, and still are, not so valid (e.g., for adolescents to inhibit growth, and for cattle and chickens to increase their growth and market value). All the anecdotal reports in the literature claimed that DES was effective, indeed a "wonder drug" (Bell 1989).

Simultaneously, in the late 1940s and early 1950s, there were randomized controlled trials of DES that consistently showed it to be ineffective in preventing reproductive wastage, and possibly harmful in some cases (Dieckmann et al. 1953). Estrogens had been shown to increase the incidence of tumors in rodents as early as 1919, and synthetic estrogens were even more powerful carcinogens than natural estrogen (Loeb 1919; Shimkin and Grady 1940). Despite these negative reports, doctors continued to prescribe DES, and its usage only slowly declined. It is always much more difficult to stop a treatment than it is to start one. At a national gynecologic conference, Dieckmann et al. (1953), from the Chicago Lying-in Hospital, reported negative results in 1,000 normal-risk pregnancies using DES, with matched controls. The Smiths responded that DES was never meant to be a "panacea." Another doctor said that he could not act on these new findings and discontinue DES because of his "civic loyalty" to his training in Boston and to the Smiths (Dieckmann et al. 1953). Thus rational data are not always sufficient to influence opinion, even among well-educated doctors. The conviction and commitment of the Smiths was more compelling to a majority of people than was a well-documented, clinical trial by respected scientists.

Newer reproductive technologies recapitulate many of these features of the DES story. They offer new hope to couples who want babies. The scientists who develop and introduce these new techniques are, understandably, very enthusiastic about their methods; their stories of wanting to give childless couples a baby are appealing to the public. The relatively few positive results are highlighted in newspaper headlines and photographs of "test-tube babies," while the personal and financial costs of these procedures, as well as the low success rates of in vitro fertilization, are minimized. A technique such as in vitro fertilization was first developed for women with blocked tubes. Indications have now broadened to include almost every infertile couple: those with female factors, male factors, and unexplained infertility (Corea 1985). To have the power to create life and to make women happy is very seductive; these wishes linger even when the hard statistics do not support the advance propaganda. The wish on the part of both physicians and parents to find the newest way to increase fertility is so powerful that it is often difficult to do adequate trials.

The DES experience also demonstrates that it is impossible to assess all the consequences for risk in the short range. Many of the DES sequelae did not begin to appear until years later when those exposed in utero reached puberty. The estimated 10 million individuals exposed to DES still live with the potential for further unfolding of the DES story.

Late Reproductive Tract Consequences of DES

The long-term effects of DES were first noticed in 1970 when seven young women came to the Massachusetts General Hospital with vaginal clear cell adenocarcinoma. This cancer, heretofore unknown in women younger than 70 years, was traced in six cases of seven to DES that the mothers of these young women had taken during their pregnancies. DES was thus the first transplacental carcinogen to be identified. The FDA issued a drug alert that notified all United States physicians to discontinue the use of DES in pregnancy. By 1970, DES had been used for pregnancy treatment in every country of the world except Denmark and Finland, where its usage was specifically prohibited. As of June 1985, 519 cases of vaginal clear cell adenocarcinoma had been listed with the International Registry for Research on Hormonal Transplacental Carcinogenesis of the University of Chicago; 60% of the cases have a documented history of maternal DES use prior to the 17th week of pregnancy and another 12% used some other hormone or medication (U.S. Department of Health and Human Services 1985). The cancer is not dose related, and the risk is present for those whose mothers took only a few doses of DES as well as for those who took the entire high-dose regimen. The estimated risk for exposed daughters through age 34 is 1:1000 (Melnick et al. 1987). Not all investigators concur with this association, and an epidemiologic reappraisal was published by McFarlane et al. (1986).

The cancer risk for DES-exposed persons has not been as dramatic as was initially feared (Hadjimichael et al. 1984). However, the cancer story continues to unfold; there is reason to suspect that as the mothers and daughters reach the age at which other estrogen-related tumors occur, they will develop more of these cancers than will their peers. For example, mothers who took DES appear to have a 1.4 relative risk of developing breast cancer compared to matched controls (Greenberg et al. 1984). DES daughters now in their 30s are reporting a higher incidence of squamous cervical and vaginal dysplasia (Robboy et al. 1984). DES sons seem to have a higher incidence of testicular tumors. In those tumors that have a high incidence in the general population, it is difficult to detect the additional risk factor from DES. Vaginal cancer was such an unusual form of tumor that even a small number of cases constituted a glaring epidemic.

Cancer has been only one of the consequences of DES usage. Fertility decrease has been experienced by two-thirds of DES-exposed offspring. Men have lower sperm counts and anomalous sperm. Women have difficulty conceiving a child, have difficulty maintaining pregnancies beyond the second trimester, and are at greater risk for premature births. Of the women whose mothers took DES, 90% have deformities of the uterus and cervix. They have more trouble using contraceptives because they may not tolerate intrauterine devices or diaphragms and do not want to take hormonal contraceptives. Adenosis (mucus-bearing tissue in areas of the vagina and cervix that usually has squamous cells) produces a lot of discharge and contributes to infection, requiring cautery or other treatment. Menstrual irregularities are common. In addition, there is the need for early and regular gynecologic examinations to detect and treat these conditions. These examinations must begin at menarche or even earlier in those who are symptomatic. The frequent gynecologic interventions themselves become additional risk factors for infertility. Gynecologic reports have attributed added infertility to post-laparotomy adhesions, conization, wedge resection, dilatation and curettage (D&C), endometrial biopsy, myomectomy, cesarean section, and hysterosalpingography (Apfel and Fisher 1984).

The newer reproductive technologies present additional risks as well as opportunities, and the risks are impossible to calculate fully. What we see from DES is that problems continue to emerge into the next generation. Reproductive tract sequelae continue, as in the several cases of malformed children born to DES daughters where the uterine deformity might have been responsible for the "grandchild" problem.

Late Nervous System and Emotional Consequences of DES

Additionally it now appears that DES, as an in utero hormone that crosses the placenta to the developing fetal brain, had an effect on the sexual dimorphic development of the central nervous system. Whereas naturally occurring hormones are inactivated by alpha-fetoprotein, synthetic hormones are not; DES binds to estrogen receptors in the fetal brain and changes the ratio of circulating estrogen to androgen. DES tends to serve as an androgenizer for the genetic female offspring who, in some studies, show more "tomboy" behavior in childhood and more assertiveness and aggression on psychological testing. For males exposed to DES, there is a feminizing influence; higher rates of homosexuality and bisexuality and fewer marriages seem to be correlated with uterine DES exposure. These effects have been studied by Meyer-Bahlburg and Ehrhardt (1986), who have been attempting to separate out the multiple variables determining sexual behavior to explore the effect of uterine hormones. Temporal lobe epilepsy and migraine are overrepresented in the DES-exposed population.

Vessey et al. (1983) conducted a follow-up survey of general practitioners who did not know which patients had been exposed to DES. They reported a significant increase in many psychiatric conditions among the DES-exposed offspring. The study design eliminated the bias of personal and familial concern. Significant increases in prevalence were found for depression, anxiety, and phobias; anorexia, addiction, and alcoholism were somewhat more common. The mothers who were subjects in the original DES trial that formed Vessey et al.'s sample had not received DES for any particular purpose, certainly not for reasons of psychiatric instability that could explain the findings as related to anything other than DES itself. A case report of schizophrenia in young men with no family history attributed their psychosis to their DES exposure (Katz 1987).

The above physical, reproductive, and neurologic effects are just part of the aftermath of DES. The emotional anguish suffered by those exposed to DES is impossible to quantify. Gutterman et al. (1985) studied DES mothers in an elegantly controlled study and showed residual lowered resilience around family crises. Shafer et al. (1984) studied the self-concept in 25 DES-exposed daughters and age-matched controls (16–30 years old) in a family planning clinic; they used a combination of self-esteem measures and interview. Those exposed to DES showed an overall positive sense of themselves, but had significantly more defensiveness, nurturance, and affiliation. When drawing themselves, they tended to obscure or omit body parts, especially sexual characteristics. The majority had experienced some health problem, and significantly more of the DES daughters (32% versus 8%) felt badly about themselves when they felt unhealthy.

The long-term emotional sequelae of this reproductive technology are largely underappreciated and are a central focus of our book: *To Do No Harm* (Apfel and Fisher 1984). DES is a paradigm for other reproductive technologies in this respect as well. The DES experience thwarted all of the wishes that went into its development and widespread usage. One of the natural responses to thwarted wishes is the development of new techniques to provide the same hope for those very same wishes—the urge to create life, make babies, and master nature. Thus further progress occurs, but the new techniques can repeat the same history.

Implications for Psychotherapy

We became interested in DES when we saw young women in our analytic psychotherapy practices who were DES daughters, and we found that the DES experience had had a profound effect on them. The DES experience was a lens through which they saw their lives and their relationships with doctors, mothers, boyfriends, lovers, husbands, and children. They had feelings and fantasies about DES that were connected to their own view of their prenatal experience and their own anticipation of motherhood. They were continually anxious about their bodies and had realistic concerns about gynecologic conditions and treatments.

DES was a quiet trauma. Yet the whole gamut of experiences usually associated with trauma has been seen in the aftermath of DES. Insults inflicted by DES are social and personal, external and internal, public and private, sudden and enduring. Emotional responses range from denial to mature integration in all parties concerned: researchers, physicians, mothers, children, and the community in general. DES and other reproductive technologies produce trauma in unique ways. They are related to sexuality and fertility, to the past and the future, and to the intimacy of the mother-child relationship. One of the most disturbing features of the DES experience is its isolating nature: the usual sources of help—mother and doctor—are unwittingly the sources of pain. The ultimate sources of help became the objects of blame, rage, grief, and sadness. The trauma of the DES experience follows from violations of feelings and relationships that are intensely private and based in the most essential expectations of trust. The obstetrician who is trained to deal with the simple and natural problems that occur in pregnancy does not expect to be the source of disasters. Reproductive care of a mother is never intended to poison the reproductive capacity of her offspring.

Psychotherapeutic work with DES daughters and mothers reveals an experience somewhere between a natural disaster and a bad dream where safe relationships appear menacing. The transference to the therapist is colored by the actual experience the DES-exposed person has had with that other doctor who said, "You can trust me; these pills are best for you and your baby." The unnatural substance of DES touched the most natural process, an area that has traditionally been intimate and untouchable. Exposure for the DES patient has a meaning connected to the frequent exposure of the physically intimate areas, and the pain, humiliation, and anxiety connected to those examinations. The analytic posture on the couch may be more difficult to assume than for other comparably neurotic individuals because of the associations to the gynecologic examination. Many character flaws and difficulties will be discussed in the metaphor of DES, which becomes a major reference point. One patient had a series of dreams about bodily disintegration and fears of having acquired immunodeficiency syndrome (AIDS); after some discussion in therapy, she said, "I don't have AIDS, I have DES!" which made new sense to her of her fears and permitted more open discussion of her realistic concerns about her DES status.

The new reproductive technologies also impinge on these private arenas, and the emotional trauma is great and subtle. DES mothers and daughters who openly express their fears, anxieties, and anger, which are appropriate responses to trauma, seem to adapt well. Women who remain isolated and who repress their feelings tend to have more disturbed body images and to develop psychosomatic symptoms.

The DES experience also led to major disruptions in the gynecologist-patient relationship; it violated the deep unspoken bond of trust between doctor and patient. Mothers have felt especially guilty, but have tended to protect their doctors by assuming responsibility themselves or by projecting blame away from the doctors onto the drug companies or the FDA. Daughters have tended to blame their mothers' obstetricians and thus spare their mothers. Mistrust of doctors makes for difficulties in the necessary ongoing gynecologic care. Doctors have tended to act defensively, to deny the causal relationship of DES to the problems seen, or to minimize their own responsibility. Doctors' withdrawal from patients only exacerbates the pain already experienced by those who suffer the trauma of DES.

Unlike their patients, physicians have responded to DES with little guilt and self-blame. Few have complied with the American College of Obstetrics and Gynecology directive to attempt actively to contact exposed female offspring to provide needed examination and information. Fear of lawsuits is not sufficient explanation for this puzzling lack of response; in fact, DES litigation is almost entirely directed at drug companies.

Patients report more distress at the physicians' blasé attitude than at the DES exposure itself. Doctors' defenses are manifested in their apparently nonchalant attitudes. The aftermath of DES is not the happy childbirth situation that attracted young obstetricians. The DES experience after all exemplifies the deepest fears of physicians: the fear of making mistakes; of failing in the eyes of peers and younger colleagues; of being criticized, regulated, and sued. It elicits feelings of helplessness and powerlessness in the face of uncertain, chronic, and unremitting illness, often in young people from families similar to their own. The usual distancing maneuvers of blaming the victim do not work. Physicians often prescribed DES for their own wives; doctors' wives and doctors themselves are well represented among the recipients of reproductive technology. Physicians are heavily represented in the population of older affluent women seeking to have children after many years of delay for career development. Success in the medical profession as physicians does not prepare at all for the experience of being a patient. If anything, knowing the possibility of error makes the doctor who is a patient even more defensive and anxious. This trauma comes close to home.

Consultation

Discussions between psychiatrists and gynecologists can be useful in this area of reproductive technologies. Ideally, this consultative relationship will be a collegial one in which the psychiatrist has input into early discussions of cases considered for noncoital reproduction. These consultations provide an opportunity to discuss ethical and emotional issues before embarking on expensive procedures. For instance, if a woman has had children removed from her care because of neglect and has had a tubal ligation and now wishes to become pregnant through in vitro fertilization, should the program consider her and her partner as potential candidates? This seemingly extreme example is offered because it produced heated debate between disciplines. The gynecologist felt the in vitro fertilization should be available to any couple where there are tubal problems precluding pregnancy and that to deny this couple would be "playing God." The psychiatrist felt that the woman's wish to become pregnant again needed to be acknowledged, but that she had not been able to cope with previous children, and it would be "playing God" to offer her the hope and possibility of pregnancy under these circumstances. The team was able to decide to evaluate the woman carefully before doing the in vitro fertilization. During the evaluation, without her partner, she revealed that she was trying to have a baby for this new man, and that she "wouldn't mind being pregnant, but don't really want another kid." The program was able to offer her a face-saving way to say to her husband that she had applied and tried, but did not meet the criteria.

The concern to heal has two major components: the innovative/active and the conserving/passive. Modern medicine with its crucial reliance on extreme technical competence and its close links to biological research and discovery strongly emphasizes the innovative/active component. There is a consistent devaluation of the conserving/passive component that is traditionally seen as the merely nontechnologic, feminine, caring characteristic. Doctors on the hospital frontier are very concerned with innovation and with the approval of their colleagues and tend to use newer methods sooner. The danger of this rapid, sometimes premature usage of new techniques is that simpler, more obvious, and less dangerous solutions may be overlooked. One example of the premature reach for high technology is the finding of one study of couples coming for in vitro fertilization (Fagan 1986). These couples showed a high incidence of sexual dysfunction and just plain ignorance about sex; sexual education allowed some of these couples to get pregnant the "old-fashioned" way.

Lessons From the DES Story

Lessons to be gleaned from the DES experience for the newer reproductive technologies are manifold. The basic moral imperative—"to do no harm"—is more important than "to do good" and must be heeded by all caretakers. In the DES example, doctors had the best intentions and wanted "to do good." Researchers and patients also had good intentions, as did the FDA. Everyone shares responsibility in our view and no one party was to blame. The lesson here is that disasters will occur even with such good intentions from all sides. Every party must be prudent and cautious, especially around reproductive technologies where many are prone to distort realities and will cast a new treatment in the most hopeful light and minimize its negative dimensions. New discoveries always have a honeymoon phase when the excitement of the investigator, the charisma of the clinical researcher, and the specialness of the first patients all combine to make the results look favorable (the so-called Hawthorne effect). It is wiser to wait and to test adequately, even if that means delays for some people. The wish to have a baby makes people desperate and willing to take risks. This desperation should not be reinforced by overly zealous researchers. When a treatment works for one group, the tendency is to expand use to more and more groups; however, what may be indicated in a limited population need not apply to everyone.

We have learned from DES that it is impossible to assess completely the long-term effects of a single pill, not to mention a complicated treatment involving several drugs, machines, and exposures to ultrasound, X rays, surgery, and anesthesia. The effects are on the woman receiving the treatment and on the unborn fetus, effects that may well continue to unfold over a lifetime and beyond. How is it possible ever to get adequate informed consent when it is not possible to inform anyone of all the later sequelae? Is informed consent ever informed enough? It is difficult enough to be honest and complete regarding just physical consequences. How is it ever possible to judge the sense of loss of bodily function and the loss of trust in essential relationships such as took place in the DES experience? We can speculate that similar losses occur in the use of other reproductive technologies. The mere listing of procedures and prescription drugs cannot begin to suggest or encompass the pain of a couple going through in vitro fertilization and their sense of loss when no pregnancy occurs (80–90% of the time), or when a pregnancy does take place and then miscarries. Potential gains are always easier to assess, and we naturally wish to emphasize such gains, which are more immediate and real (especially a baby) than to look at the dark side of major losses.

Pressures from the public, the drug companies, medical research, and government all contribute to producing more technologic innovation. We have seen in the DES story how everyone wanted this drug and welcomed it. The same is true with other technologies. There is a continual forward thrust to innovate, to cure, to solve the riddles of infertility by technical manipulation. Objective and independent evaluation of the new techniques, although essential, is very difficult. Who can and should be a powerful balancing, tempering voice? Early intervention can modify a treatment regimen before its popularity takes hold. Sometimes it takes only one person. Frances Kelsey noted the presence of limb deformities from preliminary reports on thalidomide in European journals and intervened to prevent its distribution in the United States. We learned that even with the overwhelming evidence of the carcinogenicity of DES, some of the drug's early users and supporters still deny its causal relationship to cancer and claim that the cancer is due to viruses or even to masturbation (Karnaky, cited in Gillam and Bernstein 1987)!

Human passions run strong when it comes to human reproduction. It is almost impossible for anyone to be totally objective. Therefore, ongoing dialogue and a consensus reached on relative risks and benefits are necessary. The discussions must include the possible benefits of refusing such treatments and choosing adoption or even deciding not to parent directly. Early in the DES story, negative reports about its ineffectiveness were not heeded adequately. Personal loyalties and professional allegiances caused physicians to ignore the conclusions of well-designed studies that might have halted the use of DES in pregnancy almost 20 years before the vaginal cancer epidemic did so. If new research disputes popular practice, these new results must be validated and heeded. It takes enormous effort to reverse a treatment once it has become established.

DES has taught us that people can endure a trauma quietly, that they can heal, and that they will bear scars that are there to be seen by those who can stand to look. The trauma of DES has been compounded by caretakers who do not give adequate credence to the emotional aspects of these reproductive techniques. Excessive and intrusive techniques always bring with them a sense of violation. As with other traumatic events, those people who express their feelings do better psychologically in the long run than the so-called good patients who are compliant and unquestioning.

Failed treatments such as DES have effects on caregivers that are hard to detect because the effects are subtle and because doctors have, by nature and training, well-defended characters. The feelings of failure may get transformed and transferred to bigger and more elaborate techniques and more dogged insistence on the validity of a procedure even if it has failed many times. Doctors in our personal and professional lives must learn to cope with uncertainty. The feeling that one is useful even if playing a supportive, noninstrumental role is a crucial, too-neglected part of most medical education.

Lewis Thomas (1971) defined technology in three parts: 1) the human technology of the patient-doctor relationship, which means standing by, being there as in the continuing work of psychotherapy, a kind of relationship that is needed more in infertility work; 2) the pseudotechnology of the high tech, the fancy and expensive things we devise to attack problems when we do not know the real cause or an effective treatment; and 3) real technical treatments, such as penicillin for strep throat, that are simple, inexpensive, elegant, and specific. It is the quest for this third category that must be continued. Basic research into infertility is needed. Ironically, a treatment like DES may have slowed research on miscarriage, and a procedure such as in vitro fertilization may delay more basic research into the reasons for unexplained infertility.

Following the DES fiasco in the mid-1970s, one gynecologist summed up the impact of DES by saying that "no obstetrician/gynecologist and no patient would ever again blindly take any treatment for granted!" While this view was probably overly optimistic, we believe that DES presents many lessons that we need to remember lest we repeat the same mistakes again and again.

References

Apfel RJ, Fisher SM: To Do No Harm: DES and the Dilemmas of Modern Medicine. New Haven, CT, Yale University Press, 1984

Bell SE: Technology in medicine: development, diffusion and health policy, in Handbook of Medical Sociology, 4th Edition. Edited by Freeman HE, Levine S. Englewood Cliffs, NJ, Prentice-Hall, 1989, pp 185–204

Corea G: The Mother Machine: Reproductive Technologies From Artificial Insemination to Artificial Wombs. New York, Harper & Row, 1985

Dieckmann WJ, Davies ME, Rynkiewicz LM, et al: Does the administration of diethylstilbestrol during pregnancy have therapeutic value? Am J Obstet Gynecol 66:1062–1081, 1953

Direcks A: Has the lesson been learned? the DES story and IVF, in Made to Order: The Myth of Reproductive and Genetic Progress. Edited by Spallone P, Steinberg DL. New York, Pergamon, 1987, pp 161–165

Dodds EC: The practical outcome of recent research on hormones. Lancet 2:1318–1320, 1934

Fagan P: Sexual functioning and psychological evaluation of IVF couples. Paper presented at ASPOG meeting, Philadelphia, PA, April 4, 1986

Gillam R, Bernstein BJ: Doing harm: the DES tragedy and modern American medicine. The Public Historian 9:57–82, 1987

Greenberg ER, Barnes AB, Resseguie L, et al: Breast cancer in mothers given diethylstilbestrol during pregnancy. N Engl J Med 311:1393–1396, 1984

Gutterman EM, Ehrhardt AA, Markowitz JS, et al: Vulnerability to stress among women with in utero diethylstilbestrol (DES) exposed daughters. J Human Stress, September 1985

Hadjimichael OC, Meigs JW, Falcier FW, et al: Cancer risk among women exposed to exogenous estrogens during pregnancy. Journal of the National Cancer Institute 73:831–834, 1984

Katz DL: Psychosis and prenatal exposure to DES. J Nerv Ment Dis 175:306–308, 1987

Loeb L: Further investigation on the origins of tumors in mice: internal secretion as a factor in the origin of tumors. Journal of Medical Research 40:477ff, 1919

McFarlane MJ, Feinstein AR, Horwitz RI: Diethylstilbestrol and clear cell vaginal carcinoma: reappraisal of the epidemiological evidence. Am J Med 81:855–863, 1986

Melnick S, Cole P, Anderson D, et al: Rates and risks of DES-related clear-cell adenocarcinoma of the vagina and cervix: an update. N Engl J Med 316:514–516, 1987

Meyer-Bahlburg HF, Ehrhardt AA: Prenatal DES exposure: behavioral consequences in humans. Monogr Neural Sci 12:90–95, 1986

The New York Times, April 22, 1988

Robboy SJ, Noller KL, O'Brien P, et al: Increased incidence of cervical and vaginal dysplasia in 3,980 diethylstilbestrol-exposed young women. JAMA 252:2979–2983, 1984

Shafer M, Irwin CE, Adler NE, et al: Self-concept in the diethylstilbestrol daughter. Obstet Gynecol 63:815–819, 1984

Shimkin MD, Grady HQ: Carcinogen potency of stilbestrol and estrone in strain C3H mice. Journal of the National Cancer Institute 1:119–128, 1940

Smith OW: Diethylstilbestrol in the prevention and treatment of complications of pregnancy. Am J Obstet Gynecol 56:821–834, 1948

Smith GV, Smith OW: The prophylactic use of diethylstilbestrol to prevent fetal loss from complications of late pregnancy. New Engl J Med 241:410–412, 1949

Thomas L: Notes of a biology watcher: the technology of medicine. N Engl J Med 285:1366–1368, 1971

U.S. Department of Health and Human Services: Report of the 1985 DES Task Force. Washington, DC, U.S. Department of Health and Human Services, Public Health Service, National Institutes of Health, 1985

Vessey MP, Fairweather DVJ, Norman-Smith R, et al: A randomized double-blind controlled trial of the value of stilbestrol therapy in pregnancy: long-term follow-up of mothers and their offspring. Br J Obstet Gynecol 90:1007–1017, 1983

Chapter 5

The Gynecologic Perspective

Christine L. Cook, M.D.

In the summer of 1978, the scientific world was amazed and delighted to hear of the birth of the first "test-tube baby." This and other recent scientific accomplishments have changed the way we think about reproductive capabilities. The fact that a baby can now be produced without the "normal" anatomic coupling, the fact that "abnormal" fetuses can be identified early, and the fact that the potential exists to manipulate the actual genetic content of gametes or embryos confound those of us who grew up accepting limits to what could be done to help others have a child.

A description of some of these techniques, including what they may mean to a couple, follows. The concept of "helping" needs to be redefined as we shove aside old barriers, reevaluate the concept of what is natural, and replace it with the unlimited possibility of what might be possible.

Technology of the 1980s

In Vitro Fertilization

After 10 years of intense effort on the part of a scientific team working with many loyal patients, the first child was conceived in vitro, returned to her mother, and delivered some 9 months later. The team's early efforts had been confounded by an ectopic gestation and a pregnancy that ended in a spontaneous abortion. Thanks to the persistence of couples in Dr. Patrick Steptoe's practice, work continued until Louise Brown was born (Steptoe and Edwards 1978).

Today, centers around the world work with thousands of couples in an effort to reproduce this original success. More than 5,000 infants have been born as a result of these efforts. Many centers have yet to have a success; well-established programs report the likelihood of achieving a full-term pregnancy to be 15–20%. Of all the women who are taken to an operating room to have oocytes removed, only one in six will have a live child 9 months later (Medical Research International 1988).

The in vitro fertilization process is complex and requires cooperation and understanding among the physician, the nursing and laboratory personnel, and the couple. This process usually begins with a consultation between the physician and the interested couple. Sometimes a client relationship already exists, but usually this is not the case. Therefore, such a relationship must begin at the time of the first interview, in addition to the sharing of much new information. Many infertile couples present with a long history of care: multiple laboratory tests, operative procedures, and innumerable office visits. These couples usually will have a broad understanding of the reproductive process, at least insofar as it involves their own case. Others will have been told at a single encounter that their anatomy makes conception impossible. Their understanding may be more limited.

Contact.   The first encounter must include general information about reproduction as it applies to the specific couple's infertility. It must also cover the process of in vitro fertilization per se. Finally, an assessment of the physician by the couple and vice versa will take place as they decide whether and how they will best work together. Often a nurse will be included in this consultation. The nurse can serve as a source of additional information and as a liaison with other team members throughout the process.

Procedure.   Although a few of the most well-known programs in the United States have long patient waiting lists, couples can usually begin treatment within 3 months of a contact visit. Treatment typically is initiated at the time a menstrual period begins. The woman comes to the center for baseline information about her hormonal and anatomic status. Serum estradiol, follicle-stimulating hormone, and luteinizing hormone are measured and an ultrasound of the pelvis often is done. If these parameters are satisfactory, as they usually are, a drug will be used to induce the maturation of multiple follicles in the ovaries. Generally, this medication is injected during daily office visits or by a family member trained to administer the drug. After 3 or 4 days of treatment, patients begin a series of daily visits to the in vitro fertilization center to measure serum estradiol and to evaluate the ovaries with ultrasound. The medication dose is adjusted based on the results of these tests. Usually patients are treated for 8–10 days.

For some couples, the regimen may become even more complex. A gonadotropin-releasing hormone agonist may be needed by women who do not respond well to the superovulation regimen described previously. Daily subcutaneous injection of the agonist is begun in the luteal phase and continued for 1–2 weeks until ovarian estrogen production is fully suppressed. The agonist is continued throughout the period of ovulatory drug use. Despite the use of this agent, 10–40% of cycles are canceled prior to retrieval because ovarian response has been too slow or too rapid.

Once estradiol and ultrasound evidence suggests nearly ripe oocytes, human chorionic gonadotropin is injected to mimic the physiologic luteinizing hormone surge. Retrieval is timed for approximately 34 hours later. Oocytes are retrieved either via laparoscopy or ultrasound. The method depends on the equipment of the center, the training of the physicians, and, to a lesser extent, the condition of the woman (certain ovaries are accessible only by one or the other approach due to scar tissue formation).

When the oocytes are removed, they are assessed for maturity and placed in an incubator. Mature oocytes are inseminated about 6 hours after retrieval; immature ones, 12–24 hours later. Semen samples may be collected prior to coming to the center for the retrieval or at the center after the retrieval is complete.

The day after insemination, fertilization usually can be determined by laboratory personnel. Typically, the preembryos are assessed again 48 hours after retrieval and should show division into about four cells; 80–90% of women will have preembryos to return. At this stage, they are returned to the uterus using a catheter passed through the cervix into the uterine cavity. Patients report that this procedure feels similar to having a pap smear done. Patients are asked to lie quietly for several hours after the return and to limit their activity for a day or two. Most centers have women return sometime in the luteal phase for laboratory assessment of hormone production. A pregnancy test usually is done 14 days after the retrieval.

Even if this test is positive, celebration should be deferred until an ultrasound, 3–4 weeks after the original procedure, confirms cardiac activity of an intrauterine pregnancy. Early pregnancy loss among these women is high; spontaneous abortions occur in 25% and ectopic pregnancies in about 5% of those for whom the pregnancy test has been positive initially.

Experience.   Most couples entering an in vitro fertilization treatment cycle will have spent large amounts of time and money pursuing their goal of reproduction. Anger is a familiar emotion, along with guilt and despair. Men and women want to know why they have been singled out to suffer in this way. Are they "bad"? Is this punishment for past events? Should they have chosen another life-style, partner, physician? Should they have listened to parents about not getting involved with this or that individual? Did that abortion as an adolescent make them sterile? Would another doctor, for the first operation, have prevented tubal dysfunction? Such questioning can become endless and pointless. However, certain specific answers may be quite valuable. For example, information on future pregnancy outcome among women with voluntary abortions can be provided. Descriptions of surgical procedures used in good faith 10 years ago, which are no longer "state of the art," can be provided. The role of "just relaxing and not thinking so much about getting pregnant" can be discussed, although little concrete data are available.

Identifying the agenda and working with the patient toward constructive action is part of the infertility team's job. Eventually a sense of readiness to move on, in this case to in vitro fertilization, may be reached. At this point, most couples realize that they have reached the last "moment" in their search. This may magnify the intensity of the experience for them. Throughout the in vitro fertilization treatment cycle there are points of possible "failure." Stimulation may not go well, so oocytes are not retrieved. Oocytes may look fine but not fertilize. Good embryos may be placed in the uterus, but pregnancy occurs only in one of six couples. For the other five couples who do not succeed, the whole cycle of information gathering begins again. What went wrong? Did they err somehow? Did the in vitro fertilization team not do their best work? Should another cycle be attempted? At another center? Minor adjustments in protocol or simply repeating the process will result in pregnancy for some individuals. Unfortunately, the value of these second, third, and fourth attempts is difficult to predict. If it is economically feasible, the couple usually will be encouraged to make three or four attempts. This is a fairly arbitrary recommendation, as there is limited information on the value of additional cycles. Couples who do become pregnant undergo an average of one and a half in vitro fertilization treatment cycles.

Completion.   Although an occasional couple can afford to travel and "shop" for other centers in a potentially endless pattern, for most, the last in vitro fertilization treatment cycle at the original center will be the end of their quest for a child. Exit interviews at this time may be valuable to complete the information gathering about why pregnancy has not occurred as well as to direct those involved to counselors or support systems. Unfortunately, many appointments are not kept; centers, not wishing to harass people, let the ball drop, and no further contact occurs.

New Considerations

A variety of extensions and adaptations have been used with the above protocol. Some changes are simply a part of the quest for improved pregnancy rates and outcome. Others are designed to include couples who previously have not been considered in vitro fertilization candidates.

Gamete intrafallopian transfer (GIFT).   Most common among the technique adaptations are varying the time of gamete/preembryo return. The extreme of this approach is GIFT, a procedure applicable only for women who have at least one open fallopian tube (Asch et al. 1986). In the GIFT procedure, the maturity of the oocytes is assessed immediately in the operating room; then these eggs and sperm, which were prepared in advance of the surgery, are placed into the peritoneal (ampullary) end of the tube through a catheter. Currently, this is done transabdominally through a laparoscope, but work is progressing on a transuterine technique for this placement under ultrasound observation.

Variations of this theme include the return of newly fertilized (uncleaved) oocytes into the uterus or through the uterus into the tube (Yovich et al. 1988). Some centers have worked with a "vaginal incubator" system in which eggs and sperm are initially placed in the vagina, removed a day or two later to assess development, and then returned to the woman.

Donor gametes.　For the woman who does not produce oocytes, two possibilities exist. Another woman—friend, relative, or unknown in vitro fertilization patient being treated at the same center—may agree to be stimulated, have oocytes removed as described above, and have all or some of these fertilized with the sperm of the patient's husband. These "donor eggs," once cleaving, can be returned to the patient as preembryos or returned to the tube with the partner's sperm in a GIFT procedure (Asch et al. 1988).

Another avenue for the woman who does not make eggs is in vivo fertilization. A female volunteer receives the ovulation-inducing drugs or is closely followed to monitor her time of spontaneous ovulation. This woman is inseminated in the periovulatory period with the sperm from the infertile woman's partner. A few days later, early embryos are flushed from the uterine cavity of the volunteer and placed in the uterus of the patient. Occasional success has been reported with this technique (Buster et al. 1983). When the patient has no uterus, the embryo is left in the uterus of the volunteer (surrogate mother) and allowed to develop there. Pregnancies occur much more often in this latter situation.

Changing Indications

Historically, these techniques, except for GIFT, have been reserved for couples in whom the fallopian tubes are closed, the uterus is absent, or the ovaries are not working. However, the persistence of infertile couples with other diagnoses has expanded the empirical use of these procedures. This results in pregnancy rates that vary from center to center, as well as among the different diagnoses. Success has been quite low for couples when sperm production is of a very poor quality, but surprisingly good when endometriosis has been diagnosed or when no specific infertility factor has been identified (Navot et al. 1988).

"Fertility" Drugs

Some ovulation-inducing agents have been used for nearly 30 years, and statements about their efficacy and side effects can be made. Other agents have been developed only recently; therefore, generalizations about them are less precise.

Clomiphene Citrate

In 1960, the first reports appeared about a drug that was associated with consistent ovulation and some pregnancies in infertile women with hormonally active ovaries (Tyler et al. 1960). These women with chronic anovulation syndrome, also known as Stein-Leventhal disease or polycystic ovarian syndrome, are well estrogenized, often obese, and occasionally hirsute, and have demonstrable follicles in their ovaries. Unfortunately, the hypothalamic-pituitary-ovarian axis does not function normally, thus ovulation and vaginal bleeding are erratic (Goldfarb 1977; Mills and Mahesh 1986; Rebar 1984).

Clomiphene citrate is an antiestrogen that acts by binding estrogen receptors in the hypothalamus, giving the pituitary the impression of a hypoestrogenic state. The pituitary responds by secreting follicle-stimulating hormone, thus inducing systematic follicular development in the ovaries (Kerin et al. 1985). Although this almost always results in oocyte release and subsequent menstruation, the antiestrogenic effects of clomiphene citrate are felt at other levels of the reproductive system (Adashi 1984). These and other less well understood processes reduce the pregnancy rate to less than 50%.

Side effects are uncommon: symptoms of hypoestrogenism occur in 10–20% of patients; transient ovarian cysts, in 5%; and multiple pregnancies, almost always twins, in 5% (Gysler et al. 1982). These effects almost never necessitate treatment, but sometimes are unpleasant enough to discontinue the drug.

The majority of anovulatory women have some form of chronic anovulation syndrome, are estrogenized, and will therefore ovulate when given clomiphene citrate. Other anovulatory women have hormonally inactive ovaries and produce little or no estrogen, and will therefore not respond to the antiestrogen action of clomiphene citrate. Abnormalities in these patients range from ovarian failure per se to pituitary and hypothalamic malfunction (Kletzky et al. 1975). Some women are untreatable, but others will respond to treatment of the specific hypothalamic or pituitary disorder or to specialized ovulation-inducing medication.

A very small group of infertile women undergo early or premature menopause. For these women there is no possibility of genetically "mothering" a child. Nonetheless, with a uterus in place, they are logical candidates for egg or embryo donation. The expense and limited availability and success of donation programs make this an uncommon solution. Most of these women will never carry a child.

Human Menopausal Gonadotropin

Other women will respond well to the use of human menopausal gonadotropin (Pergonal) for ovulation induction. For 20 years this urinary extract of luteinizing hormone and follicle-stimulating hormone has been administered to mimic the usual pituitary secretion of these hormones (Schwartz et al. 1980). Precise administration is difficult. Despite careful monitoring, as outlined above for in vitro fertilization patients, there is a high incidence (25%) of multiple pregnancy. Usually twins are the result, but as many as nine embryos are known to have been conceived. A second side effect is that of hyperstimulation. Some women will develop large luteal cysts on their ovaries, resulting in pain, fluid shifts, and, very rarely, thromboembolic disease and death. Approximately 1 in 50 human menopausal gonadotropin cycles will result in brief hospitalization for monitoring and care of hyperstimulated women (Diamond and Wentz 1986).

For women with chronic anovulation syndrome, the decision to use clomiphene citrate usually is not a difficult one because of the limited side effects encountered. On the other hand, hypoestrogenic women have a much more difficult choice—between the potentially serious side effects of human menopausal gonadotropin listed above and childlessness.

Gonadotropin-Releasing Hormone

The improved understanding of the relationship between the hypothalamus and the pituitary has fostered the development of gonadotropin-releasing hormone as an ovulation-inducing agent (Schriock and Jaffe 1986). When administered daily, gonadotropin-releasing hormone shuts down pituitary release of luteinizing hormone and follicle-stimulating hormone. However, when administered at 60- or 90-minute intervals in low doses, a release similar to the physiologic release of the gonadotropins occurs. Ovulation, usually of a single egg, is the result. Pulse dose can be increased if superovulation is the goal. Monitoring does not have to be intense for women on low-dose regimens; often periovulatory urine sampling for spontaneous luteinizing hormone release is sufficient.

Ideally, gonadotropin-releasing hormone is administered intravenously, necessitating the use of a pump worn on the body affixed to an intravenous line in the forearm. Local irritation of the intravenous site is uncommon, and infection is rare, but not all women are comfortable with the idea of wearing this apparatus for 1–3 weeks (Corenblum et al. 1985).

With both human menopausal gonadotropin and gonadotropin-releasing hormone, women who previously have been accustomed to low estrogen levels may have side effects associated with excess estrogen. These are not medically serious, but may be quite unpleasant (e.g., headaches, breast tenderness, abdominal bloating, and swelling of the hands and feet).

Successful pregnancy occurs in about half of anovulatory patients using these medications. The rate of ectopic pregnancy does not appear to be increased, whereas spontaneous abortion may occur slightly more often than in the general population. Prematurity, as a result of multiple pregnancy, and its attendant perinatal morbidity and mortality are significant concerns.

Changing Indications

As with in vitro fertilization, the original indications for the use of ovulation-inducing agents have been markedly expanded. They now include the larger group of women with other infertility diagnoses as well as those in whom a diagnosis has not been made (Dodson et al. 1987; Kemmann et al. 1987; Melis et al. 1987).

Approximately one in three of these normally ovulating women will become pregnant with a few months of human menopausal gonadotropin therapy. (Comparable information is not available for gonadotropin-releasing hormone.) At least this many women would also become pregnant with no treatment at all over a period of several years (Lam et al. 1988). How to balance risk against time is a difficult question for most couples.

Surgical Approaches to Infertility

Endoscopic instruments for viewing the pelvic contents have been used for many years; however, the development of improved optics and light-generating equipment has made such visualization common in the last 20 years. Laparoscopy, which allows direct assessment of the peritoneal aspect of the uterus, tubes, ovaries, and adjacent surfaces, has been the most frequent procedure. Unfortunately, general anesthesia and a small abdominal incision(s) are usually required. The small but real risk of laparoscopy is associated with these features (Musich and Behrman 1982).

The recent development of the hysteroscope has provided a view of the endometrial surface of the uterus (Valle 1980). This procedure can complement laparoscopy or be used independently in some cases without general anesthesia or abdominal entry. Finally, scopes are being developed to assess the interior of the fallopian tubes directly. These appear to offer information in addition to that currently available via hysterosalpingogram (contrast radiography) (Shapiro et al. 1988).

Each of these endoscopes is being adapted for use as a therapeutic as well as a diagnostic instrument. Direct cauterization, heat endocoagulation, and a variety of laser beams can be directed into the peritoneal or uterine cavities to destroy or remove scar tissue, endometrial implants, and uterine abnormalities. Risks, which appear to be low, apart from those associated with the diagnostic procedure itself, are related more to user training and experience, as expected. Endoscopic procedures are associated with less hospitalization, with less physical discomfort and recovery time, and thus with lower costs than the previously popular laparotomy procedures. The advantage for fertility and/or pregnancy outcome, however, is not yet well established. The difficulty of performing randomized trials and the impossibility of blind trials is obvious.

The role of sequential operative procedures for infertility patients is also unclear. The concept is sound: after a reparative procedure, before additional scar tissue has an opportunity to vascularize, a follow-up laparoscopy is performed to remove early, filmy adhesions. However, until the efficacy is established, patients cannot balance the risk of a second operative procedure against an unknown gain (Trimbos-Kemper et al. 1985).

The Personal Experience

Infertility is perhaps best defined as the failure of an individual to achieve a pregnancy within his or her own elective time frame. When this goal is not met, information gathering is always useful, and medical care may be appropriate.

Information Gathering

Information can be obtained from several sources. Informally, couples talk with friends or family members. Sometimes these individuals are well informed through their own experience or employment. In other cases, feelings may be shared, but knowledge not advanced.

Libraries and bookstores now offer a variety of printed material on this subject. Some is too technical to be useful to any except the most sophisticated consumer; other work can be a guide to almost anyone. Information about health events or medications that may predispose one to infertility, definitions of "normal" for the menstrual cycle, or directives about the timing of coitus may help. In some cases, couples will become pregnant; in others, couples may realize that medical help will be necessary.

Changing Medical Care Team

Some general practitioners and many obstetrician gynecologists will be able to offer useful advice, begin an evaluation, and/or initiate treatment. When pregnancy occurs, these actions have been sufficient. However, when infertility persists, some couples will benefit by referral to physicians with special training in reproductive endocrinology and infertility. Board subspecialization in this area has been formalized for physicians caring for women but not for men. Certain internists and urologists with an interest in the field have expanded their education and experience to include the care of the infertile male. The American Fertility Society is a voluntary, special-interest group of physicians, scientists, and nurses who work with infertile patients. No specific credentials are required for membership.

A move toward more specialized care may be suggested and encouraged by the primary care physician. Sometimes, however, it is initiated by the patient without support from this provider. In such circumstances, patients may feel disloyal or guilty, as well as insecure, as they move from the familiar to the uncertain. The ideal time for such a move is not always clear. However, the use of medications that require special monitoring (e.g., human menopausal gonadotropin) or the need for surgical procedures not traditionally included in residency training programs in obstetrics and gynecology (e.g., laser laparoscopy) may dictate the need for a different physician. Uninvolved physicians, such as psychiatrists, may provide advice and "legitimacy" at this juncture (Daniluk 1988).

"Public" Exposure

The move from physician A, often a local person, shared with sisters and friends, to physician B in a different town or practice is usually the time at which the quest for fertility becomes "public," at least in the sense that it becomes known among close friends and family. In addition, such a move often involves an increased expenditure of time and money as more technical services are incorporated. Days off from work, avoiding usual leisure activities due to budgetary adjustments, and the increasing strain or optimism as care proceeds are other changes that may be noticeable. Explanations can range from factual sharing with close friends to various "excuses" offered to distract the boss or a nosy co-worker. Such duplicity intensifies the pressure experienced by a couple.

As the infertility care continues, any privacy between the male and female partner or between either of them and the physician, nurse, nursing assistant, laboratory technician, and even the billing clerk and appointment desk personnel is lost. This sense of complete exposure through frequent examinations, reviews of ovulation temperature charts designed to include statements about date and time of coitus, and/or monthly semen evaluations (for inseminations) places an immeasurable burden on those involved. Introspective questions arise. Have we been "good?" Have we done the "right" thing? Did our bodies cooperate?

The strain is increased by the inability of the health care team to answer such questions in many situations. Help can be provided, however, by continued education and instruction as well as by assisting in nonjudgmental language, replacing words like *good* and *right* with technical statements.

Simultaneously, however, the emotions that have led to such statements should be addressed.

As one month follows another, with stress adding to disappointment and as each menstrual period signals another point of grief or loss (the child who would have been conceived in April 1988 and would have been born next January—you know, the one I imagined would have your blue eyes and my dark hair—is now irrevocably lost), decisions must be made.

Decision Making

Infertile individuals are now able to enter into a high technology phase of care. Unfortunately, the more complex the medical program, the less likely it is to succeed. Although this generalization does not apply to every situation, it is a good adage to keep in mind. Furthermore, many of the most elaborate techniques for pregnancy assistance do not increase the long-term probability of a pregnancy occurring; they simply shorten the time period in which this will happen. Finally, the exact role of some treatments in some patient groups has not been evaluated scientifically, making any statement about efficacy only a best guess.

In the face of such confusion, discouragement, and stress, many couples are well advised to take periodic breaks in their active pursuit of a child. This need not in any way be construed as failure or giving up. In fact, however, by deciding not to continue care for a period of time (e.g., the summer months), the couple will feel that they are giving up or losing the specific child that might have been conceived during each one of those cycles. Also they worry about disappointing their spouse, whose need for a rest may not yet be as intense. There is even a concern about "letting down" the health care team who has been working so diligently along with them. Permission to take this time off can be provided with only a few words at the appropriate time.

This time-off decision is a temporary one and, by definition, easier than decisions about stopping or not "moving up" the treatment ladder. Setting goals for time, financial, and personal commitment is valuable for the couple, who by now have been involved for some months or years. Several criteria can be used for making such decisions. Perhaps the simplest is time. If a procedure (e.g., intrauterine insemination) has never been known to be successful after 9 months of use, one can stop at that point. If 90% of the pregnancies that result will occur during the first five cycles, that may be a reasonable time goal. Unfortunately, this information is only now being worked out for the most intense procedures, such as in vitro fertilization.

Financial goal setting may be more difficult even though more facts are available. One can learn specifically what three cycles of superovulation or two cycles of in vitro fertilization will cost. Financial habits and discipline differ greatly from one couple to another. Some will not embark on any treatment plan until the money is set aside. Others will borrow or hope to earn more or receive support from other sources (e.g., family). This is an area in which the infertility specialist is unlikely to have had any appropriate training, but should encourage patients to seek advice elsewhere.

Closure

The most difficult time in this entire process is the moment when a couple agree that they will stop actively seeking medical treatment. Sometimes, financial resources are exhausted, making further treatments impossible. More often, the choice is truly that, a choice. A decision must be made. Perhaps at the outset the pair agree not to subject each other to major physical risks. In that case, they may decide to stop when the remaining alternatives involve major surgery for the woman or fertility drugs that could result in multiple pregnancy with risks to the infants. Perhaps there was an early decision to stop when the odds became "very unfavorable." Usually, at the point when this earlier plan is invoked, much energy has already been expended and objectivity is harder to come by.

For some, this final decision means that they will never have their own biological child; for others it means that the possibility exists, but the odds are not in their favor. Often this decision is initiated by one or the other involved person, who must then convince her or his partner. This is not an easy process for either individual. Each has struggled to obtain the elusive goal, devoting enormous time and energy to the process. These women and men are not "quitters," yet now is the time to stop. Now they must not only maintain their own conviction, but also share it with the physician and others with whom they have worked. Sometimes they slip away, simply not keeping a visit and then not making another appointment. But closure means to complete the process. If possible, a mutual agreement with shared permission giving will allow this goal to be met.

Much disappointment peripheral to the specifically involved couple must be dealt with. The physician may have not wanted them to "give up." An anxious parent will not want to hear that his or her oldest son will not be passing on the family name. Another parent will have to continue knitting for someone else's grandchildren. Friends will move on to their circle of activities that include shared complaints about late-night feedings, school committees, or camping with everyone's kids.

Nevertheless, the relief of finally knowing what will happen and the certainty of being in charge of one's body, one's daily schedule, and one's sexuality brings a comfort that has been absent for a long time. Simply adjusting to this daily freedom occupies the mind for awhile. Sooner or later, however, one begins to look beyond the habit of counting time from one menstrual cycle to another.

Most of us grow up with changing views about what our profession will be, where we might live, what sort of a person we wish to marry, how many children we will have—note, how many is the question, not if. Changing this image of ourselves as a parent requires work. All of those things we were going to do with our time, the sharing of oneself—biologically, physically, and emotionally—for which we have prepared, must now be replaced. For some women and men, the transition to job- or hobby- or friend-orientation occurs slowly but steadily. For others, it may seem impossible that any new self could be as valuable, as worth being, as that parent-self that cannot be. Therapy is often necessary to make this shift (Schroeder 1988).

Outside Support for Decision Making

Throughout the infertility process, decisions must be made individually and agreed on and carried out jointly. There may be couples who can move through the decisions with ease, relying on their own personal resources. Many, however, will require and/or benefit from outside support. Such support may be necessary to provide legitimacy in the face of a health care team that is encouraging the couple to continue this search for a biological child or in the face of family and friends who aren't ready to accept this finality.

Support may also be valuable as the couple once again return to a life in which they can choose—choose what to do with their time, choose how to spend their money, and choose when to express themselves sexually. For some, the infertility process has lasted the majority of their adult/married life. Changed identities (the nonparent self) and new patterns of action and interaction will need to be developed. Change requires work and time, both of which are now available.

Summary

Although the birth of Louise Brown signaled a new era in reproductive technology, the fact remains that only one of two couples seeking infertility care will be successful. The quest for a child can be arduous, involving not only the couple, but their extended support environment and a large team of health care personnel. If the goal remains elusive, more and more complicated procedures and medications will be invoked. Complicated psychosocial and physical demands will be encountered. Although formalized support systems are almost always constructive, therapeutic intervention will sometimes be necessary for processing this major life event.

References

Adashi EY: Clomiphene citrate: mechanism(s) and site(s) of action—a hypothesis revisited. Fertil Steril 42:331–344, 1984

Asch RH, Balmaceda JP, Ellsworth LR, et al: Preliminary experiences with gamete intrafallopian transfer (GIFT). Fertil Steril 45:366–371, 1986

Asch RH, Balmaceda JP, Ord T, et al: Oocyte donation and gamete intrafallopian transfer in premature ovarian failure. Fertil Steril 49:263–267, 1988

Buster JE, Bustillo M, Thorneycroft IH, et al: Non-surgical transfer of in vivo fertilised donated ova to five infertile women: report of two pregnancies. Lancet 2:223–224, 1983

Corenblum B, Mackin J, Taylor PJ: Ovulation induction and pregnancy in women with hypothalamic amenorrhea treated with intermittent gonadotropin-releasing hormone. J Reprod Med 30:736–740, 1985

Daniluk JC: Infertility: intrapersonal and interpersonal impact. Fertil Steril 49:982–990, 1988

Diamond MP, Wentz AC: Ovulation induction with human menopausal gonadotropins. Obstet Gynecol Surv 41:480–490, 1986

Dodson WC, Whitesides DB, Hughes CL Jr, et al: Superovulation with intrauterine insemination in the treatment of infertility: a possible alternative to gamete intrafallopian transfer and in vitro fertilization. Fertil Steril 48:441–445, 1987

Goldfarb AF: Polycystic ovarian disease: clinical considerations. J Reprod Med 18:135–138, 1977

Gysler M, March CM, Mishell DR Jr, et al: A decade's experience with an individualized clomiphene treatment regimen including its effect on the postcoital test. Fertil Steril 37:161–167, 1982

Kemmann E, Bohrer M, Shelden R, et al: Active ovulation management increases the monthly probability of pregnancy occurrence in ovulatory women who receive intrauterine insemination. Fertil Steril 48:916–920, 1987

Kerin JF, Liu JH, Phillipou G, et al: Evidence for a hypothalamic site of action of clomiphene citrate in women. J Clin Endocrinol Metab 61:265–268, 1985

Kletzky OA, Davajan V, Nakamura RM, et al: Clinical categorization of patients with secondary amenorrhea using progesterone-induced uterine bleeding and measurement of serum gonadotropin levels. Am J Obstet Gynecol 121:695–703, 1975

Lam S-Y, Baker G, Pepperell R, et al: Treatment-independent pregnancies after cessation of gonadotropin ovulation induction in women with oligomenorrhea and anovulatory menses. Fertil Steril 50:26–30, 1988

Medical Research International, The American Fertility Society Special Interest Group: In vitro fertilization/embryo transfer in the United States: 1985 and 1986 results from the national IVF/ET registry. Fertil Steril 49:212–215, 1988

Melis GB, Paoletti AM, Stigini F, et al: Pharmacologic induction of multiple follicular development improves the success rate of artificial insemination with husband's semen in couples with male-related or unexplained infertility. Fertil Steril 47:441–445, 1987

Mills TM, Mahesh VB: Gonadotropin secretion in polycystic ovarian syndrome and related diseases. Seminars in Reproductive Endocrinology 4:109–113, 1986

Musich JR, Behrman SJ: Infertility laparoscopy in perspective: review of five hundred cases. Am J Obstet Gynecol 143:293–303, 1982

Navot D, Muasher SJ, Oehninger S, et al: The value of in vitro fertilization for the treatment of unexplained infertility. Fertil Steril 49:854–857, 1988

Rebar RW: Gonadotropin secretion in polycystic ovary disease. Seminars in Reproductive Endocrinology 2:223–230, 1984

Schriock ED, Jaffe RB: Induction of ovulation with gonadotropin-releasing hormone. Obstet Gynecol Surv 41:414–423, 1986

Schroeder P: Infertility and the world outside. Fertil Steril 49:765–767, 1988

Schwartz M, Jewelewicz R, Dyrenfurth I, et al: The use of human menopausal and chorionic gonadotropins for induction of ovulation: sixteen years' experience at the Sloane Hospital for Women. Am J Obstet Gynecol 138:801–807, 1980

Shapiro BS, Diamond MP, DeCherney AH: Salpingoscopy: an adjunctive technique for evaluation of the fallopian tube. Fertil Steril 49:1076–1079, 1988

Steptoe PC, Edwards RG: Birth after the reimplantation of a human embryo. Lancet 2:366, 1978

Trimbos-Kemper TCM, Trimbos JB, van Hall EV: Adhesion formation after tubal surgery: results of the eighth-day laparoscopy in 188 patients. Fertil Steril 43:395–400, 1985

Tyler ET, Olson HJ, Gotlib MH: The induction of ovulation with an anti-estrogen. Int J Fertil 5:429–432, 1960

Valle RF: Hysteroscopy in the evaluation of female infertility. Am J Obstet Gynecol 137:425–431, 1980

Yovich JL, Yovich JM, Edirisinghe WR: The relative chance of pregnancy following tubal or uterine transfer procedures. Fertil Steril 49:858–864, 1988

Chapter 6

Legal Implications of the New Reproductive Technologies

Colleen K. Connell, J.D.

New developments in reproductive medicine and technology are forcing a reevaluation of the traditional legal concepts that governed family life and procreation. Such procedures as in vitro fertilization, cryopreservation of fertilized ova, artificial insemination, and reproductive services contracts, including "surrogacy" arrangements,[1] now allow the separation of the genetic, gestational, and coital components of reproduction. Historically, with the exception of restrictions relating to marriage, lawmakers have attempted to impose few restrictions on attempts by people to procreate. However, simultaneously with this new technology has come the call for government to restrict severely, or at least regulate, its use.

Not surprisingly, the legal system, which is primarily reactive, did not establish an anticipatory legal framework within which to resolve the inevitable conflicts arising from the use of such technology. Accordingly, there is some uncertainty as to the legality of certain procedures. This uncertainty may lead infertile couples to forgo use of certain reproductive procedures and also may lead physicians to avoid developing or offering such procedures.

Given the increased recognition of fertility problems suffered by many people, as well as the development of medical technologies to treat these

My appreciation is extended to Darryl DePriest, Elizabeth Thompson, and Jeff Cusic for their assistance in preparing this article.

problems, the impetus to use these technologies has become overwhelming. The legal system's response to this pressure is beginning to take shape. This response includes the extension of existing legal principles to new factual situations and the enactment of new laws specifically designed to deal with reproductive technology.

This chapter will include a discussion of the parameters, both constitutional and statutory, within which state and federal governing bodies regulate the development and use of new reproductive technologies. The impact of these principles on the rights of patients and the rights of physicians, including psychiatrists, also will be discussed. Finally, specific legislative attempts to regulate this technology and the resolution of conflicts resulting from the use of the technology will be analyzed in an attempt to provide some guidance as to the optimal role of psychiatrists in legal situations involving new reproductive technologies.

The United States Constitution

The United States Constitution, which explicitly guarantees freedom from many different types of governmental restrictions, unfortunately does not explicitly guarantee any right of reproductive freedom or any right to use technology and medical techniques either to procreate or to avoid procreation.[2] Notwithstanding the absence of express constitutional protection, there is strong societal and legal support for allowing individuals to make decisions about procreation without undue governmental interference.[3] At least two separate doctrines—the personal right of privacy and a limited right of scientific inquiry—have developed in the case law interpreting the Constitution and should protect people who wish to use reproductive technology to attempt to have a child and physicians who wish to develop that technology and offer it to their patients. However, neither of these doctrines has explicitly dealt with any psychiatric or psychological implications of either procreation or the decision not to procreate.

Development of the Right to Privacy

The right of privacy is a fundamental right vested in the individual. Over the past 60 years, the United States Supreme Court has ruled that the Constitution protects the individual from governmental invasions into personal decision making in matters that greatly affect the most intimate details of their lives. The development of this doctrine has been among the most positive and significant in modern constitutional law. The zones of personal privacy protected from unwarranted governmental interference include decisions about whom one chooses to marry;[4] the use of contraceptives by married couples,[5] and by unmarried people;[6] and whether a woman chooses to have an abortion.[7]

Reproductive or procreative freedom is not limited to the right to avoid conception or childbirth. The freedom to procreate is "one of the basic civil rights of man."[8] The importance of this right to procreate has been emphasized repeatedly by the Supreme Court:

> The decision whether or not to beget or bear a child is at the very heart of this cluster of constitutionally protected choices. That decision holds a particularly important place in the history of the right of privacy, a right first explicitly recognized in an opinion holding unconstitutional a statute prohibiting the use of contraceptives, . . . and in the contexts of contraception, . . . and abortion. . . . This is understandable, for in a field that by definition concerns the most intimate of human activities and relationships, *decisions about whether to accomplish or to prevent conception are among the most private and sensitive* [emphasis added]. If the right of privacy means anything, it is the right of the individual, married or single, to be free of unwarranted governmental intrusion into matters so fundamentally affecting a person as the decision whether to bear or beget a child.[9]

If the constitutional right of privacy protects the decision to reproduce coitally because of the social and biological importance of being a parent, it should also protect decisions to procreate with the assistance of reproductive technology, including noncoital techniques.[10] The United States Supreme Court, however, has not ruled on whether the constitutional right to privacy includes the use of reproductive technology in an attempt to procreate. As discussed more extensively below, decisions by lower federal and state courts, which are of less precedential authority, have reached conflicting decisions. One state supreme court has ruled that the right to privacy does not encompass such reproductive techniques as surrogacy;[11] another state supreme court suggested that the right to procreate, even when assisted through technology, is protected.[12] In a closely related area, a lower federal court concluded that the right to privacy extends to protect the right of individuals to use the most technologically advanced medical techniques to help make decisions about reproduction.[13]

Whether and to what extent the Supreme Court ultimately will extend the right of privacy to protect the use of reproductive technology is uncertain. Some legal theorists assume an unduly cramped view of the Constitution and would interpret it to protect only those rights explicitly enumerated within the text of the document, such as the right to freedom of speech. These critics contend, among other things, that by striking down laws that regulate private decision making on issues regarding home and family, the Supreme Court has intruded into the broad realm of authority that state legislatures usually are afforded to regulate matters pertaining to health and welfare. Several members of the Supreme Court unfortunately appear to agree with this school of thought.[14]

Given the Supreme Court's July 1989 decision in *Webster v. Reproductive Health Services*, it is not inconceivable that the Supreme Court would cut back on the privacy doctrine or decline to extend it. In *Webster*, a bitterly divided Court upheld a Missouri law restricting abortion. At least four members of the Court—Rehnquist, White, Kennedy, and Scalia—expressed great dissatisfaction with existing Supreme Court decisions protecting reproductive privacy and suggested a willingness to accept as constitutional more state restrictions of this right.[15] Given the *Webster* decision, it is not unlikely that any cutback would come in a case involving abortion rights, given the continued push in that direction by anti-abortion advocates and the Court's announcement that it would review three more abortion cases during its 1989–1990 term. However, judicial restriction of the right to procreative and sexual privacy might easily involve a case attempting to extend the right to privacy to protect a range of private conduct,[16] including the development and use of reproductive technology.

A decision by the United States Supreme Court to curtail the right to procreative freedom would profoundly and negatively disrupt the existing state of the law. Millions of people would be left without any constitutional protection from legislation restricting their attempts to use medical and technologic means to help them become parents. Many more people could be subjected to laws should states choose to enact them, restricting the use of some or all contraceptives[17] and restricting other parental choices—all rights persons have freely exercised *without* undue governmental interference. The legal and human costs of such a decision obviously weigh against such a restriction of the right of privacy.

Development and Scope of the Right of Scientific Inquiry

The second legal doctrine that arguably protects the development of reproductive technology from unwarranted governmental restriction is the constitutional right to practice one's profession and to secure knowledge. As long ago as 1923, the Supreme Court recognized that this right had constitutional dimensions, holding that the due process clause of the Fourteenth Amendment to the United States Constitution protects the right of a person to engage in the occupations of life and to acquire useful knowledge.[18] In *Roe v. Wade*,[19] and its companion case of *Doe v. Bolton*,[20] the Supreme Court recognized that physicians have a constitutional right to practice medicine freely according to the highest medical standards without arbitrary governmental restraints. Similarly, the Court has recognized that the First Amendment protection of free speech includes the right to receive information freely.[21] Research directed at developing new reproductive technology should be protected by the First Amendment right of inquiry;[22] the administration of that therapy to consenting patients should be protected by the physician's right to practice in accordance with medical standards and the patient's right of procreative privacy.[23]

The case law delineating the scope of the physician's right to practice or to engage in the development of new techniques provides a less compelling basis for protecting freedom than does the right of individual procreative privacy. Although the constitutional underpinning of both rights flow, in part, from a theory that the Constitution protects a certain right to be left alone, courts have not construed expansively this right of research and inquiry.

Perceived Governmental Interests in Regulating Use and Development of Reproductive Technology

The fact that the Constitution protects a certain sphere of procreative activity does not mean that all regulation of this subject will be ruled unconstitutional. For years, government has regulated the use of oral contraceptives and the intrauterine device so as to protect the health of the woman.[24] Likewise, government constitutionally can enact laws to fund certain reproductive options, such as childbearing, and decline to fund alternatives, such as abortion.[25] Thus government has no obligation to finance the reproductive choices people have made. To justify laws that restrict privately exercised and privately funded reproductive choices, however, the government first must demonstrate that the regulation is needed to further a compelling governmental interest. Once a legitimate regulatory interest has been established, the government also must show that the regulation is so carefully drawn that it regulates in the least restrictive manner possible.[26]

One interest articulated as potentially compelling enough to justify some regulation of reproductive technology is the need to protect women (and occasionally men) from the risks entailed by use of several of the technologic processes, including the risk of emotional or psychological harm.[27] The need to protect a patient's health is a compelling enough reason to support narrowly drawn regulations so long as the government can prove that the regulation actually advances the patient's health.[28]

The second ostensible interest in regulating reproductive technology is the desire to protect the embryo or any child ultimately born of such reproductive technology from possible physical risks inherent in the procreative technology itself or from the psychological risks of being born as a result of technologically assisted reproduction. This "interest" gained enhanced importance recently because in *Webster*, Chief Justice Rehnquist, writing a plurality opinion in which three other justices joined, suggested that concern for the embryo or fetus could justify restrictions at all points after fertilization of the ovum had occurred. Obviously, advancing this interest in a way that restricts the use of technology risks protecting the embryo or ultimate child at the expense of the constitutional rights of the woman and the man who are attempting to procreate. To ensure people the broadest scope of reproductive freedom, only regulations actually proved to protect the fetus or child, without materially restricting the persons attempting to procreate, should be sustained.

Finally, many attempts to restrict reproductive technology focus on the perceived need to protect certain values, such as the sanctity of human life and maintaining traditional methods of procreation through the nuclear family.[29] These interests, while certainly deserving of serious thought and discussion, should not be considered compelling enough to justify substantial governmental restrictions on reproductive technology. Restrictions based on moral values often advance the ethical concerns of a few members of society at the expense of the fundamental reproductive rights of others. As noted recently by the American Fertility Society, such a result overlooks the plurality of our society.[30]

Given the importance of procreation to individuals, and the assistance that technology can provide for people with fertility difficulties, attempts to restrict reproductive technology should meet with very careful scrutiny.[31] The Baby M case,[32] involving the attempted enforcement of a "surrogacy" contract, presents for such scrutiny nearly all of the competing interests discussed above: the reproductive privacy interests of the man and woman attempting to have a child; concern for any child ultimately born; and the moral concerns of "tampering with nature." This case is a helpful model for analyzing the interface between the legal system and psychiatrists and psychologists in the area of reproductive technology.

Attempts to Regulate or Restrict Development and Use of New Reproductive Technologies

Dispute Engendered by the Baby M Case

Although the roots of surrogacy arguably can be traced to biblical times, recent surrogacy agreements seem to have precipitated a great deal of controversy and proposed regulation.[33] The legal community is sharply divided on the issue of whether the constitutional right of privacy protects the right to enter into a reproductive services contract,[34] and, if so, whether that right to privacy carries with it a corresponding right to enforcement of the contract by the legal system. The Baby M case honed this legal conflict.

This case involved a dispute between the genetic father (William Stern) and the genetic and gestational or surrogate mother (Mary Beth Whitehead).[35] Mrs. Whitehead contracted to be artificially inseminated with Mr. Stern's sperm, bear a child, and relinquish that child to Mr. Stern and his wife, Elizabeth. After the baby was born, Mrs. Whitehead changed her mind and sought to maintain her parental rights.

A legal battle ensued, with the trial court finding that surrogacy contracts were legal and that the right of persons to enter into such contracts was protected by the constitutional right of reproductive privacy.[36] In finding that surrogacy was protected, the trial court in the Baby M case ruled that "if one has the right to procreate coitally, then one has the right to reproduce non-coitally. If it's the reproduction that is protected, then the means of reproduction also are to be protected."[37] The trial court found that Mrs. Whitehead had breached the contract and also found that not only the terms of the surrogacy contract but also the best interests of the child dictated that permanent custody be awarded to the Sterns.

The prestigious New Jersey Supreme Court in the Baby M case reversed the trial court and ruled that the constitutional right of privacy neither protected the right to enter into a surrogacy contract nor required that custody of the child be resolved according to the terms of the contract. The New Jersey Supreme Court found that "the parties' right to procreate by methods of their own choosing cannot be enforced without consideration of the state's interest in protecting the resulting child. . . ."[38] The state supreme court equated surrogacy with baby selling and, with surrogacy thus characterized, ruled that it was violative of both the New Jersey adoption law and public policy. Such contracts, found the court, result in an inevitable conflict of fundamental interests: the father's interest in procreation, the gestational mother's interest in the companionship of the child, and the best interests of the child.

Psychiatric consultation and testimony played an important role in the Baby M case, not only in the personal lives of the parties but also in the legal analysis employed by the trial court and by the New Jersey Supreme Court. After determining that Elizabeth Stern risked aggravating her multiple sclerosis were she to attempt to bear a child, the Sterns had explored many procreative options.[39] The Sterns finally concluded that a surrogacy arrangement best advanced their hope to have a child.

Elizabeth Stern sought professional counseling after the diagnosis of multiple sclerosis was made; it is not clear whether either of the Sterns received professional mental health care during the time they entered into the surrogacy contract. The surrogacy contract prepared at the behest of the Sterns, however, reflects the importance the Sterns placed on psychiatric care—Mrs. Whitehead was to submit to a preinsemination psychiatric evaluation for which Mr. Stern would pay.[40] The purpose of the examination was to determine whether Mrs. Whitehead would be able to relinquish the child on its birth. This requirement appears to be a standard provision of many surrogacy contracts.[41]

Testimony by mental health professionals—psychiatrists, psychologists, and social workers—formed a key part of the evidence heard by the trial court in the Baby M case. These witnesses testified about the mental state of the parties, the psychological risks surrogacy posed, and whether the best interests of the child required that either the Sterns or Mrs. Whitehead be given custody. After hearing this testimony, the trial court determined that custody should be awarded to the Sterns, whom the judge found to be stable loving people who "have expressed a willingness, and a history of obtaining professional help, to address the child's unique problems."[42]

Although the New Jersey Supreme Court reversed part of the trial court's decision and ruled that the surrogacy contract was invalid and could not be enforced, it too afforded great weight to the psychological testimony, especially concerning the stability of the competing parties and their parenting skills, that had been relied on by the trial court in concluding that custody should be given to the Sterns. In rejecting Mrs. Whitehead's claim for custody, the New Jersey Supreme Court found that she would be too controlling a parent, and that Baby M's "prospects for a wholesome independent psychological growth and development would be at risk."[43] In reaching this decision, the court clearly was troubled by Mrs. Whitehead's "contempt for professional help," even though it recognized that professional counseling is not a sine qua non of good parenting.[44]

Although both the trial court and the New Jersey Supreme Court relied on testimony by mental health professionals, this case exposed the legal and mental health issues lurking behind the use of new reproductive technology. Neither court finally resolved all of these issues. Future litigants and legislative bodies still face many of the problems identified in the Baby M case.

In Vitro Fertilization, Artificial Insemination, and Other Techniques

Other technological methods designed to help people with fertility problems—especially embryo transfer and artificial insemination—potentially present legal issues very similar to those raised by the surrogacy debate. With respect to artificial insemination and embryo transfer, difficult issues of custody could be raised: the artificial insemination donor might, at some future time, wish to assert parental interests in any child produced through artificial insemination; the couple providing the genetic material for the embryo that is transferred to another woman's uterus for gestational purposes may find themselves confronting a custody battle similar to that seen in the Baby M case; or a dispute might arise over the future of a frozen embryo and a battle for the "custody" should the couple providing the genetic material disagree as to its disposition or should a medical facility refuse to relinquish a frozen embryo.[45] If the artificial insemination donation was pursuant to medical protocol and anonymous, it is unlikely that a court will recognize parental rights in the donor.[46] However, if the fertility problem experienced by a couple stems from the woman's inability to carry a pregnancy rather than to produce an ovum for fertilization and the couple produces a fertilized ova that is flushed and then transferred to another woman for gestational purposes, it is not impossible that a custody battle would ensue. The issues would be slightly different than those posed in the Baby M case, however, as both members of the couple desiring the child would have a genetic link to the child, whereas the woman who gestated the child would not.

Legislative Efforts to Regulate Reproductive Services

In the wake of the Baby M controversy, bills proposing to regulate surrogacy were introduced into many state legislatures. The provisions of these bills ranged from a complete prohibition of surrogacy, such as Illinois House Bill 2101,[47] to bans on only paid surrogacy, such as Louisiana House Bill 327,[48] to bills that would provide for the recognition of a surrogacy relationship.[49] Also, House Bill 2433 has been introduced in the United States Congress and would prohibit the exchange of money for the making, engaging in, or brokering of a surrogacy contract.[50] Much of the proposed legislation, however, allows surrogacy in some form.[51]

The mental health aspects of surrogacy arrangements are of great concern and are specifically addressed in several legislative proposals. While professional mental health consultation for people considering technology-assisted reproduction often is helpful and should be encouraged,[52] important issues of individual decision making and confidentiality must be considered before any type of mandated consultation or disclosure is enacted into law. The potential problems raised by such laws, for both mental health professionals and their patients, are illustrated by a few of the bills now pending. However, before proceeding with a surrogacy arrangement, the law of the state in which the parties are contracting must be examined closely.

Illinois Senate Bill 1510, pending indefinitely before the Illinois General Assembly, specifies the terms necessary for an enforceable reproductive services contract and, as one of the requirements, mandates that the surrogate and her husband, if any, be apprised of and consent to "any medical and *psychological* [emphasis added] risks associated with the performance of the reproductive services agreement."[53] Disclosure of this information to the gestational mother herself fulfills what courts have described as the physician or mental health professional's duty to impart information that the patient has every right to expect[54] so that the patient can make an informed judgment when determining whether to consent to artificial insemination and the hoped for pregnancy, with all of its potential medical and psychological implications. Failure to advise a patient of the potential material implications of a medical procedure may give rise to a valid cause of action for lack of informed consent.[55] Requiring disclosure of psychological data certainly might help prevent situations like that in the Baby M case, where the preliminary psychological examination of Mrs. Whitehead showed that she might experience great difficulty relinquishing custody of the child.[56]

However, expanding this disclosure requirement to include persons other than the gestational mother presents many potential problems. If the gestational mother had been counseled alone by the mental health professional, disclosure without her consent, even to her husband, of information gathered from her during a confidential session seems to conflict with the mental health professional's ethical obligation to preserve the confidences of her or his patient.[57] Unwarranted disclosures of private information may give rise to a malpractice suit or a suit claiming invasion of privacy.

States arguably will attempt to justify enacting laws forcing disclosure by claiming a compelling interest in protecting children born of such agreements. However, the difficulty of predicting either the behavior of the gestational mother or the impact on any child ultimately born undercuts the persuasiveness of this justification. Alternatively, if the prospective adopting couple employed the potential gestational mother and paid her to submit to a mental health examination, there is some legal authority allowing disclosure to an employer in order to serve important societal interests.[58] The societal interests at stake here—protection of the contracting parties and the potential child—which do not rise to the level of protecting someone from serious bodily harm, should not be considered sufficiently compelling to justify forced disclosure of personal facts against the person's consent.

While mental health services should be encouraged,[59] serious civil liberties concerns are evoked by proposals that such services be required as a matter of law as a condition precedent to entering into a reproductive services contract.[60] With limited exceptions, such as testing for sexually transmitted diseases prior to marriage, the government cannot constitutionally compel competent adults to submit to medical procedures.[61] If a woman has a constitutional right to procreate through a surrogacy contract, a law mandating a psychiatric examination before she could enter into such a contract might well be considered an unconstitutional burden on her reproductive freedom.[62] Likewise, if a couple has the constitutional right to use technologically assisted reproduction, a law requiring mental health care may violate the fundamental rights of procreative autonomy and the right to refuse medical treatment or evaluation. Compelled mental health evaluations also raise a specter of concern over how these evaluations will be used. Evaluations should be used only to help people make educated and informed decisions. They must not be used to restrict parenting to only those people sharing values or life-styles mental health professionals consider acceptable.

In recognition of these civil liberties concerns, an Indiana law provides that it is against public policy to enforce any term of a reproductive services agreement that requires a gestational mother to "[u]ndergo medical or psychological treatment or examination."[63] Mental health professionals should abide by and encourage respect for the civil liberties of persons using reproductive technology. It would be painfully ironic to forgo personal privacy to use technology that is constitutionally protected under the rubric of privacy.

Role of Mental Health Professionals in Shaping Law and Public Policy Governing Reproductive Technology

Need for Precontractual and Prelitigation Services

A key issue in any reproductive services arrangement, be it for surrogacy or for a procedure such as in vitro fertilization, is establishing that informed consent actually was given before a reproductive services contract was entered into. Professional counseling to ensure informed decision making might prove critical should litigation ensue about the interpretation or enforcement of a reproductive services contract. Although the law will vary from state to state, as a general matter, informed consent is predicated on two factors: first, the patient having sufficient intellectual capacity to understand the options and the risks of the procedure being contemplated; and, second, the physician transmitting the information concerning options and risks to the patient before the patient undergoes the procedure in question.[64]

Detailing the options available to couples experiencing fertility problems is not difficult: they can opt to continue to try to conceive coitally; they can choose to undergo whatever medical or surgical technique the physician recommends; they can try to adopt a child; or they can decide to forgo their plans to try to have or raise a child. The physical risks of the reproductive procedure being contemplated, such as laparoscopy or in vitro fertilization, often can be identified and should be explained thoroughly, just as they would be for any other medical or surgical procedure.

The psychological risks of such procedures are more difficult to identify generally and must be assessed on an individual basis by the mental health professional who examines the patient; what may be an important risk to one person may not be a risk for another. Parties contemplating the use of technologically assisted reproduction, such as laparoscopy and then in vitro fertilization, might be counseled about the difficulties of having the privacy and the spontaneity of coital reproduction stripped away.

Couples considering artificial insemination by donor might be advised of any potential concerns the husband might have because he is not genetically linked to the child the wife ultimately bears. Surrogacy arrangements also present a Pandora's box of potential problems, including the problems identified above. To ensure complete disclosure of the risks, mental health professionals who evaluate the parties before a surrogacy contract is executed should consider, among other factors: 1) the parties' willingness to enter into the arrangement and that no party is being pressured to "go along"; 2) that the gestational mother is fully apprised of the risks of bonding with the child and then relinquishing the child; 3) that the gestational mother be advised of possible risks to her existing children who may not understand the surrogacy arrangement; 4) that both the gestational mother and the genetic father and his wife understand any possible psychological risks that may be posed to the child when he or she learns of his or her origins; and 5) that the wife of the genetic father knows she may experience difficulties by virtue of the fact that she may not be genetically linked to the child she is to parent and that another woman bore her husband's child.

Professional counseling should be urged before the contract is actually negotiated, with full disclosure to the person(s) counseled of every possible psychological risk of such a procedure, if the risk is material. If appropriate, voluntary disclosure could be made to other participants in the agreement. Counseling also should be available during the term of the reproductive services contract or during the time the medical technologies or procedures are being administered and, in the case of surrogacy, after the birth of the child. Professional counseling also might be beneficial in other contexts, such as situations involving the need to reduce selectively octuplet and quadruplet pregnancies that have resulted from the use of fertility drugs in the treatment of infertility.[65] An obvious but important caveat is that the informed consent determination needs to be made on the facts presented by each individual case.

Mental Health Professionals as Expert Witnesses

It is inevitable that mental health professionals will be called to testify as expert witnesses in disputes involving reproductive technology. The evidentiary rules that govern such expert testimony vary from state to state, but the rules of evidence that are applicable in federal courts serve as a reliable model for evaluating the purpose and scope of expert psychiatric testimony. As a matter of general principle, a psychiatrist, psychologist, or other mental health professional will be allowed to testify as an expert witness if his or her "scientific, technical, or specialized knowledge" will help the judge or the jury "to understand the evidence or to determine a fact at issue."[66] Before such testimony is allowed, however, the lawyer must "qualify" the mental health professional as an "expert" by demonstrating to the judge, through a series of questions asked of the witness, that he or she does in fact possess the specialized "knowledge, skill, experience, training, or education"[67] that will be of assistance at the trial. Once a mental health professional is qualified as an expert, his or her testimony is likely to reflect an opinion based on personal observations of the parties or hypotheticals concerning the subject of the dispute; or to reflect an opinion based on information or data, such as a scientifically valid study, of the type usually relied on by a mental health professional in forming opinions or conclusions.[68]

Trial court judges have a great deal of discretion in deciding whether to allow a witness to testify as an expert and in determining the extent to which the expert testimony will be relied on and credited. Judges often seem to be reluctant to weigh heavily testimony on new techniques and technologies. Accordingly, mental health professionals asked to testify in disputes involving reproductive technology should be especially meticulous in their preparation. If an opinion based on a personal consultation is required, care should be taken to examine thoroughly the person on each of the issues on which testimony is required.[69] Alternatively, if the opinion to be given is based on scientific data or studies, great care should be taken to ensure their scientific validity.[70]

Mental health professionals who do not take such care in preparing risk having their testimony excluded from consideration or risk having their testimony discredited in a bruising cross-examination by the opposing attorney. If, on the other hand, the expert testimony is thoroughly prepared, it can be most helpful in educating the judge or jury on a variety of issues, including 1) whether the parties gave informed consent to either the medical procedure at issue or the reproductive services contract; 2) whether the gestational mother or the genetic father and his wife should have custody of the child; 3) whether other terms of a reproductive services contract should be enforced; and 4) the scope of the emotional damage a party suffered as a consequence of either the medical technique or the enforcement or the breach of the reproductive services contract.

Mental Health Testimony Before Legislative Bodies

Mental health professionals also have an important role to play in educating the public at large about the new reproductive technology. New reproductive technology is often viewed with some resistance when it is first introduced, with acceptance developing only gradually.[71] Mental health professionals should actively pursue opportunities to present testimony to legislative bodies contemplating regulation of reproductive technology. Such testimony could be helpful on a number of issues, including 1) the importance of procreation to the psychological development and fulfillment of individuals; 2) the need to proceed carefully in regulation so as not to deprive persons with fertility problems of the psychological benefits of childbearing; 3) the psychological benefits, if they can be documented, of, for example, a gestational mother entering into a surrogacy contract; and 4) the psychological harms, if they can be documented, of the various reproductive technologies.

Conclusion

The law governing reproductive technology is likely to undergo a number of changes and developments in the next several years. Hopefully, the law will accommodate the legitimate needs of people experiencing fertility problems to rely on technologic advances to help them achieve what is one of the most important of all rights: the right to attempt to have a family. Mental health professionals will play a major role in helping to address societal fears about the consequences of this new technology and in educating not only the legal profession and litigants through expert trial testimony, but also society at large through testimony before legislative bodies and fact-finding commissions. Thoughtful and well-documented testimony on such issues could help produce laws and public policy that safeguard not only the right of reproductive privacy but also concerns for the well-being of the parties to such reproductive services, and any children ultimately born.

Notes

1. Surrogacy arrangements—or reproductive services contracts—are agreements pursuant to which a woman agrees to gestate and bear a child through aided conception, such as artificial insemination, for another person with the intention of relinquishing her parental rights to that child after birth. Often, the woman who gestates the child is called a "surrogate mother." However, a more appropriate and accurate description would be to refer to the woman as the gestational or birth mother. A gestational mother may donate the ovum that is fertilized and thus is both the genetic and the gestational mother. Or someone other than the gestational mother, such as the woman who is married to the man who provides the sperm, may donate the ovum for gestation by the gestational mother.

2. The United States Constitution provides the analytical foundation against which all law governing reproductive technology must be analyzed. If a right is protected by the Constitution, actions by the federal government that are found by a court to conflict with the guarantees of the Constitution have been declared unconstitutional and enjoined from enforcement by the federal courts since the early days of this country. Likewise, actions by state governments found to conflict with the Constitution are unconstitutional and unenforceable because the Supremacy Clause in Article VI of the Constitution states unequivocally that "the Constitution, and the laws of the United States which shall be made in pursuance thereof . . . shall be the supreme Law of the Land . . . any Thing in the Constitution or Laws of any State to the Contrary notwithstanding."

3. Karst K: The freedom of intimate association. Yale Law Journal 89:624, 1980

4. Loving v Virginia, 388 US 1 (1967)

5. Griswold v Connecticut, 381 US 479 (1965)

6. Eisenstadt v Baird, 405 US 438 (1972)

7. Roe v Wade, 410 US 113 (1973). But see Webster v Reproductive Services, No 88-605 (July 3, 1989). In this case, the Supreme Court upheld as constitutional a Missouri law restricting abortion. See discussion below at notes 13–17.

8. Skinner v Oklahoma, 316 US 535, 541 (1942)

9. Carey v Population Services Int'l, 431 US 678, 685 (1977)

10. See Robertson J: Embryos, families, and procreative liberty: the legal structure of the new reproduction. Southern California Law Review 59:939, 1986.

11. In the Matter of Baby M, 109 NJ 396, 537 A2d 1227 (NJ 1988)

12. Surrogate Parenting v Commonwealth ex rel Armstrong, 704 SW2d 209 (Ky

1986). See also In the Matter of the Adoption of Baby Girl, 505 NYS2d 813 (NY 1986). The decision in the Kentucky case may have been undercut by a recently enacted Kentucky law restricting surrogacy. See Ky Rev Stat Ann §199.590(3) (1988).

13. See Lifchez v Hartigan, No 82 C 4324 (ND Ill, App 26, 1990); Margaret S. v Treen, 597 F Supp 636, 673 (D La 1984) (ban on fetal research unduly limits medication information obtainable and thus deprives women of information needed to make reproductive choices), aff'd on other grounds, 794 F2d 994 (5th Cir 1986).

14. Thornburgh v American College of Obstetricians & Gynecologists, 476 US 747, 789 (1986) (White J, dissenting). In his dissent, which was joined by now Chief Justice Rehnquist, Justice White criticized the majority's interpretation of the Constitution to protect the right of reproductive privacy, noting: "A reader of the Constitution might be surprised to find that ... the text obviously contains no references to abortion, nor, indeed, to pregnancy or reproduction generally."

15. Prior to Webster, Hartigan v Zbaraz, US, 108 S Ct 479 (1987), rehearing denied, US, 108 S Ct 1064 (1988), was the Court's most recent abortion case. In the Zbaraz case, the Supreme Court again was sharply divided and, by a 4-4 vote, affirmed the decision of the lower federal court, which had ruled unconstitutional major portions of an Illinois law requiring that both parents be notified of their teenage daughter's decision to have an abortion. Justice Kennedy, who appears to be among those who would sharply curtail a woman's right to have an abortion, had not been confirmed when the Zbaraz case was argued and decided. Justice O'Connor is the swing vote on this issue, whereas Justices Brennan, Marshall, and Blackmun are strongly supportive of continuing constitutional protection for individual decisions about reproductive concerns.

16. See Bowers v Harwick, 478 US 186 (1986) (constitutional right of privacy does not extend to protect the right of homosexuals to engage in consensual sexual activity).

17. For example, the General Assembly of Illinois has enacted a law, presently enjoined, stating that should the abortion and privacy cases be reversed or modified, the General Assembly would try to return the law in the state of Illinois to its former policy of prohibiting abortion unless it is necessary to preserve the woman's life—Ill Rev Stat Ch 38, par 81-1 et seq (1987). Other provisions in this enjoined law, §2(7) and 11(3), would require a physician, under pain of criminal prosecution, to describe the intrauterine device and low-dose oral contraceptives as abortifacients rather than contraceptives.

18. Meyer v Nebraska, 262 US 390, 399 (1923)

19. Roe v Wade, 410 US 113 (1973)

20. Doe v Bolton, 410 US 179 (1973)

21. Stanley v Georgia, 394 US 557, 564 (1969)

22. See Robertson J: The scientist's right to research: a constitutional analysis. Southern California Law Review 51:1203, 1978.

23. See Andrews L: Medical Genetics: A Legal Frontier. Chicago, IL, American Bar Association, 1986, pp 50–51.

24. See 21 CFR §310.501 (federal regulations governing oral contraceptives); 21 CFR §310.502 (federal regulations governing intrauterine devices for human use for the purposes of contraception).

25. See Harris v McRae, 448 US 297 (1980); see also Webster v Reproductive Health Services, 109 S Ct 3040 (1989).

26. Roe v Wade, 410 US 113, 155 (1973). In Webster v Reproductive Health Services, several members of the Supreme Court criticized and called into question this very exacting judicial standard for evaluating restrictive state laws.

27. This may include assurance that the persons agreeing to use reproductive

technology have given a voluntary and *informed* consent to the procedure, as discussed later. See also Andrews and Hendricks: Legal and moral status of IVF/ET, in Foundations of In Vitro Fertilization. Edited by Fredricks CM, Paulson JD, DeCherney AH. Washington, DC, Hemisphere, 1987, p 312.

28. Thornburgh v American College of Obstetricians & Gynecologists, 476 US 747, 759 (1986)

29. In 1987, the Roman Catholic Church, through its Congregation for the Doctrine of the Faith, issued its Instruction on the Respect for Human Life in Its Origin and on the Dignity of Procreation. The Instruction was highly critical of new reproductive technology and concluded that noncoital reproductive techniques are morally illicit.

30. See American Fertility Society: Ethical considerations of the new reproductive technologies, Report of the Ethics Committee of the American Fertility Society in Light of Instruction on the Respect for Human Life in Its Origin and on Dignity of Procreation at 3-30 (February 1987).

31. By way of analogy, prior to Webster, almost every governmental attempt to regulate and restrict contraceptive and abortion services had been declared unconstitutional and enjoined. See, e.g., Roe v Wade, 410 US 113 (1973); Planned Parenthood of Central Missouri v Danforth, 428 US 52 (1976); Colautti v Franklin, 439 US 379 (1979); and City of Akron v Akron Center for Reproductive Health, 462 US 416 (1983).

32. In the Matter of Baby M, 525 A2d 1128 (1987), aff'd in part, rev'd in part, 537 A2d 1227 (NJ 1988)

33. Andrews L: The aftermath of Baby M: proposed state laws on surrogate motherhood. Hastings Center Report 31, Oct/Nov 1987

34. Compare Robertson J: Surrogate mothers not so novel after all. Hastings Center Report 28, Oct 1983, with Corea G: The Mother Machine: Reproductive Technologies From Artificial Insemination to Artificial Wombs. New York, Harper & Row, 1985, pp 213–249.

35. Mrs. Whitehead also was to be the genetic mother of the baby.

36. In the Matter of Baby M, 217 NJ Super 313, 525 A2d 1128 (1987)

37. In the Matter of Baby M, 217 NJ Super 313, 525 A2d 1128, 1164 (1987). The Baby M case involved a surrogate contract whereby Mrs. Whitehead agreed to be artificially inseminated with sperm from Mr. Stern and to relinquish custody of the child immediately after birth. After the baby girl was born, Mrs. Whitehead declined to relinquish custody.

38. In the Matter of Baby M, 537 A2d 1227 (NJ 1988)

39. In the Matter of Baby M, 525 A2d at 1128

40. In the Matter of Baby M, 525 A2d at 1143

41. As discussed in more detail below, few if any such contracts require the genetic father and his wife to undergo psychiatric consultation either before or after the contract is entered into.

42. By way of contrast, the trial court concluded that the expert testimony indicated that Mrs. Whitehead was impulsive and had difficulty making rational decisions in times of stress. The trial court also found that she was manipulative and would have difficulty subordinating her own needs to those of the child. In the Matter of Baby M, 537 A2d at 1259.

43. In the Matter of Baby M, 537 A2d at 1259

44. In the Matter of Baby M, 537 A2d at 1258-59

45. Such litigation was initiated in Virginia. Plaintiffs sued those in charge of an in vitro fertilization program for refusing to allow the plaintiffs to transfer their frozen embryos to an in vitro program in California in which plaintiffs were enrolled. The case ultimately settled, with the in vitro fertilization program transferring the embryo to the couple providing the genetic material.

46. See In the Matter of Baby M, where the New Jersey Supreme Court noted that

A sperm donor simply cannot be equated with a surrogate mother. The State has more than a sufficient basis to distinguish the two situations—even if the only difference is between the time it takes to provide sperm for artificial insemination and the time invested in a nine-month pregnancy—so as to justify automatically divesting the sperm donor of his parental rights without automatically divesting a surrogate mother. (p 1254)

Approximately 30 states have enacted law delineating the appropriate medical requirements for artificial insemination donation and setting the parenthood implications of insemination—Andrews L: The aftermath of Baby M: proposed state laws on surrogate motherhood. Hastings Center Report 31, 33, Oct/Nov 1987. However, if the sperm donor did not contribute the sperm anonymously and had some sort of relationship with the woman inseminated, at least one court has recognized parental rights in the donor. See C.M. v C.C., 152 NJ Super 160, 377 A2d 821 (1977).

47. Illinois House Bill 2101 provides that "[n]o person shall enter into, or participate in, any surrogate parenthood arrangement." The bill also provides that

The State of Illinois has long recognized that any form of commercialization in relation to the placement or adoption of children is immoral and contrary to the State's goal of ensuring and protecting the welfare of children. The State of Illinois also recognizes the risk of harm from the variety of disputes that may result from an arrangement under which a woman agrees to bear a child for another person, and the consequent risk of emotional harm to a child born as a result of such an arrangement.

The Utah Legislature enacted House Bill 129 in April 1989, which states that "[n]o person shall be a party to an agreement or contract . . . [to] terminate a mother's parental rights." Some state legislatures have acted to discourage surrogacy without banning it expressly by enacting statutes that presumptively place the parental rights over a child conceived through artificial insemination in the birth mother and, correspondingly, appear to terminate the parental rights of the sperm donor. See Ala Code §§26-17-21; 26-17-18 (1988); Wisc Stat §891.40; 69.14 (1988).

48. La Rev Stat Ann §9:2713 (1987)

49. Ark Stat Ann §9-10-201 (1987); 1989 Iowa House Bill 628

50. House Bill 2433, 100th Congress 1st Sess, to amend 18 USC §1822. The bill died in committee.

51. See generally Andrews L: The aftermath of Baby M: proposed state laws on surrogate motherhood. Hastings Center Report 31, 34, Oct/Nov 1987.

52. Seibel M: A new era in reproductive technology: in vitro fertilization, gamete intrafallopian transfer, and donated embryos. N Engl J Med 318:828, 833, 1988. For example, professional mental health services should be encouraged when people first consider surrogacy as a reproductive option and, should that choice be made, during the negotiation of the surrogacy contract itself. Professional consultation also is to be encouraged after the child is born—for the gestational mother and the adoptive parents, as well as for the child.

53. Illinois Senate Bill 1510, §7(d)(6). The bill does not identify what it considers the psychological risks to be.

54. See Canterbury v Spence, 464 F2d 772 (DC Cir), cert denied, 409 US 1064 (1972).

55. See Roberts v Patel, 620 F Supp 323 (ND Ill 1985). It is important to note that, as of this date, no such actions concerning the use of reproductive technology have been prosecuted against mental health professionals.

56. Unfortunately, this evaluation was never shared with either Mrs. Whitehead or the Sterns.

57. See Miles v Farrell, 549 F Supp 82, 84 (ND Ill 1982). Likewise, the Current Opinions of the Council on Judicial and Ethical Affairs of the American Medical Association dictate that

The information disclosed to a physician during the course of the relationship between the physician and patient is confidential to the greatest possible degree. The patient should feel free to make a full disclosure of information in order that the physician may most effectively provide needed services. The patient should be able to make the disclosure with the knowledge that the physician will respect the confidential nature of the communication. The physician should not reveal confidential communications or information without the express consent of the patient, unless required to do so by law.

The obligation to safeguard patient confidences is subject to certain exceptions which are ethically and legally justified because of overriding social considerations. Where a patient threatens to inflict serious bodily harm to another person and there is a reasonable probability that the patient may carry out the threat, the physician should take reasonable precautions for the protection of the intended victim, including notification of law enforcement authorities. Also, communicable diseases, gun shot and knife wounds should be reported as required by applicable statutes or ordinances. (American Medical Association: Current Opinions of the Council on Judicial and Ethical Affairs of the American Medical Association, 21. Chicago, IL, American Medical Association, 1986, p 21)

58. See generally Gelman R: Prescribing privacy: the uncertain role of the physician in the protection of privacy. North Carolina Law Review 62:255, 1984. In the context of mental health professionals, such disclosure usually is warranted only when it is needed to prevent the risk of grave bodily harm to a third person. See Tarasoff v Regents of University of California, 17 Cal3d 425, 131 Cal Rptr 14, 551 P2d 334 (1976).

59. See Seibel M: A new era in reproductive technology: in vitro fertilization, gamete intrafallopian transfer, and donated embryos. N Engl J Med 318:828, 833, 1988.

60. One provision in a bill pending before the Illinois General Assembly requires the surrogate and her husband to submit to such an examination so that the mental health professional can determine whether they are "fit persons capable of surrendering the child at birth"—Illinois Senate Bill 1510 §7(d)(6).

61. Governmental interventions involving forced intrusion of a person's body are carefully scrutinized because no right is held more sacred than the right of every individual to the possession and control of his or her own body. Accordingly, the United States Supreme Court has found unconstitutional state attempts to compel examinations of criminal suspects for the purpose of gathering evidence. See Rochin v California, 342 US 165, 172 (1952) (forcible pumping of a criminal suspect's stomach was "conduct that shocks the conscience" and that violated the suspects Fourteenth Amendment due process rights); Winston v Lee, 470 US 753, 764 n 7 (1985) (unconstitutional to remove surgically a bullet from a suspect's body against his or her will). A forced psychiatric examination as a condition to exercising a fundamental right

seems to present the same difficulties. But see National Treasury Employee Union v Von Raab, 109 S Ct 1384 (1989) (concerns of safety and national security justify drug testing of governmental employees who seek to be promoted to positions that involve interdiction of drugs or require them to carry firearms); Skinner v Railway Labor Executives' Ass'n, 109 S Ct 1402 (1989) (government's interest in regulating the conduct of railroad employees to ensure safety presents special needs beyond normal law enforcement that make drug testing a not unreasonable search).

62. Compare City of Akron v Akron Center for Reproductive Health, 462 US 449-50 (1983) (requirement that a woman undergo a mandatory waiting period to ensure that she has thought about abortion decision and ramifications is unconstitutional burden on woman's right of reproductive privacy).

63. Ind. Code §31-8-2-1(a) (1988)

64. In the Baby M case, for example, Mrs. Whitehead claimed that she did not give an informed consent to the surrogacy contract because she was not aware of all of the risks, including that of bonding with the child, incumbent in such an agreement. The trial court rejected this argument—525 A2d at 1149. Compare Hartke v McKelway, 707 F2d 1544, 1548-49 (DC Cir), cert denied, 464 US 983 (1983).

65. Evans M, Fletcher JC, Zader IE, et al: Selective first-trimester termination in octuplet and quadruplet pregnancies: clinical and ethical issues. Obstet Gynecol 71:289–296, 1988

66. Rule 702, Federal Rules of Evidence

67. Rule 702, Federal Rules of Evidence

68. Rule 703, Federal Rules of Evidence

69. In the Baby M case, the trial court did not give much weight to the psychiatrist who testified that Mrs. Whitehead had not given an informed consent to the surrogacy contract because the judge concluded that a 1-hour interview with Mrs. Whitehead was insufficient to establish such a fact. In the Matter of Baby M, 525 A2d at 1148-49. See also Goldstein v Kelleher, 728 F2d 32, 39 (1st Cir 1984) (psychiatrist not allowed to testify on whether patient gave informed consent where psychiatrist had not examined patient until 3 years after the surgery at issue and where the psychiatrist had not questioned the patient on the issue of her consent).

70. See United States v Board of School Commissioners of City of Indianapolis, 506 F Supp 657, 666 (SD Ind 1979) (court would not rely on psychological and sociological testimony about effects of desegregation because "expert" witnesses had not relied on statistical data in establishing predicate for testimony).

71. Andrews L: The aftermath of Baby M: proposed state laws on surrogate motherhood. Hastings Center Report 31, Oct/Nov 1987

Chapter 7

Second-Generation Ethical Issues in the New Reproductive Technologies: Divided Loyalties, Indications, and the Research Agenda

John D. Lantos, M.D.

There are now 24 ways to have a baby (Table 1). Six of these are currently in use: 1) so-called natural reproduction; 2) artificial insemination by donor; 3) in vitro fertilization (IVF) with embryo transfer; 4) embryo washout and transfer; 5) surrogate mothering; and 6) adoption. Ten others will probably be used in the future (Weaver and Escobar 1987).

These therapies offer powerful means for providing medical solutions to the problem of infertility. They may also be used to reduce the incidence of genetic disease, or to select desirable genetic traits in our offspring. Because the range of applications of these therapeutic techniques is so broad, and because they deal with procreation, a wide range of ethical issues arise in the actual or potential uses of these techniques.

In each of these techniques, slightly different issues may arise. For example, the ethical issues raised by surrogate mothering are different from those raised by artificial insemination by donor. Furthermore, different methods can be combined, with different ethical implications. For example, in surrogate mothering, the issues are different if the surrogate is the genetic mother of the fetus, if the ovum was donated by the prospective parent (IVF

Table 1. Twenty-four ways to have a baby

Options	Possibilities	Total
1st gamete (from female)	Wife or donor	2
2nd gamete (from male)	Husband or donor	2
Site of fertilization	Wife, in vitro, or surrogate	3
Site of pregnancy	Wife or surrogate	2
Total possibilities: $2 \times 2 \times 3 \times 2 = 24$		

with embryo transfer), or if the ovum was donated by a third woman (embryo washout and transfer).

Today's ethical dilemmas must be understood in the context of two decades of rapid scientific progress, and two decades of serious and penetrating ethical analysis. To put today's ethical issues into context, I will briefly review the relationship between the development of the therapeutic techniques and the development of ethical thought over the last 20 years. I will show how rapidly ethical norms evolved to reflect the facts as they became known through scientific progress. I will then discuss ethical problems that will require attention from psychiatrists in the decade to come.

First-Generation Ethical Issues in the New Reproductive Technologies

Edwards et al. first described the fertilization of human oocytes in vitro in 1969. Their work generated a storm of controversy, much of which was related more to the fantasies of reporters and science-fiction writers than to the facts that Edwards et al. reported. The press hailed the creation of "test-tube babies," falsely implying that these babies would grow entirely outside the body. Philosophers and theologians argued about the moral status of the fertilized ova, and of the embryos that developed. Were they people? Did they have souls? If they were not people, was their moral status different from other laboratory specimens? When did "life" begin? If research was to be carried out, from whom should consent be obtained (Walters 1979)? Proposed answers to these moral questions focused on absolute principles and tried to decide whether the work was "right" or "wrong" by weighing competing and often contradictory moral principles.

Edwards and colleagues argued, by contrast, that their work was morally justified because its goal, to help couples condemned to a life of infertility to have their own child, was morally justified and consistent with the goals of medicine (Steptoe and Edwards 1972). The only relevant ethical principles, they argued, were those that demanded that research that might enable them to reach this goal should be careful and thorough (Edwards 1985). Accordingly, they systematically evaluated the risks of the IVF process.

After they established that fertilization could take place in vitro, they showed that ova fertilized in vitro could be developed to the blastocyst stage (Edwards et al. 1970). These two preliminary achievements changed the debate from a theoretical one about test-tube babies to a practical one about the in vitro methodologies most likely to succeed and about the risks involved in each method. Questions of absolute principles receded and were replaced by technical questions about likely and unlikely outcomes. How certain could the investigators be that they would not create "monsters?" Should the benefit to the parents outweigh the risks to the child (Kass 1971)? The middle ground of the ethical dialogue began to shift, and risk-benefit analyses replaced sermons.

This shift from an ethical system that judged actions based on whether they conformed with fixed and established principles to a system that judged actions based on the desirability of the results achieved by the action mirrored the investigators' view of the ethical issues. Even they, however, felt constrained by some absolute principles. Although they felt that the safest and most scientifically useful procedure would have been extensive pre-implantation research on embryos in the laboratory, this course would have involved the disposal of some embryos. If the embryos had the moral status of human beings, this disposal could not be ethically justified. At this point, the investigators yielded to the moralists and refrained, temporarily, from experiments on human embryos.

Instead, animal experiments were carried out to see whether IVF and reimplantation resulted in "normal" or "deformed" births. Preimplantation embryos of many species were subjected to noxious agents, drugs, X rays, temperature changes, and so forth. The findings were interesting. Nature seemed to have built a fail-safe mechanism into the reproductive process. The embryos were found either to grow normally or not to develop at all. There were no "intermediates" (Steptoe 1985).

Armed with data showing that the procedure was unlikely to produce deformed babies, the investigators felt that the benefits to prospective parents outweighed the risks to prospective children, and they proceeded with attempts at IVF and embryo reimplantation in humans. The first attempts were discouraging. For 3 years, they were unable to establish a pregnancy. In 1975, an ectopic pregnancy was established, but it ended in miscarriage. Nature's fail-safe mechanisms appeared to be quite good, but progress continued, until 3 years later Louise Brown was born.

The birth of a normal baby proved that IVF was possible, but it did not prove anything about the risks and benefits of the procedure. In the circus atmosphere surrounding newsworthy medical innovations, however, determination of risks or benefits is less influential than the dramatic story of a medical triumph (DeVries 1988). Everything turns on the outcome of the first case or two. If the first human IVF baby was imperfect, arguments about benefits for infertile patients outweighing risks would have collapsed like a house of cards. As it turned out, the first baby was fine. She stimulated the development of a medical technology that will have widespread effects on both infertile patients and the rest of society.

Second-Generation Ethical Issues in the New Reproductive Technologies

The story of the development of the new reproductive technologies shows how ethical discussion and technical progress seem to take place on tracks that only occasionally intersect. Moral questions about the moral status of the embryo or the moment at which life begins, which seemed urgent in 1969, are still unanswered today. Work has proceeded without confronting them, and today these questions are largely irrelevant and seem almost quaint.

People with principle-based moral objections are left behind, while those without objections push ahead. The Vatican statement on alternative methods of reproduction condemned all noncoital reproduction as an immoral separation of procreation from coitus (NC Documentary Service 1987). It condemned research on embryos, asserting that human life begins at conception and that embryos have the same moral status as any other human being. Although nothing in the scientific work refutes this opinion, the success of that work becomes its own justification. By the end of 1983, IVF programs were in operation in 25 countries; 590 babies had already been born after 517 IVF pregnancies, and, according to one survey, there were 570 clinical pregnancies still ongoing in January 1984 (Henahan 1984). In 1986, 6,000 cycles of ovarian stimulation were performed in the United States alone. By 1987, at least 3,000 babies were born after IVF. There are now at least 160 IVF clinics in the United States, 10 of which began in 1987 (Raymond 1988).

Psychological counseling is integral to the function of IVF clinics (Berger 1980; Freeman et al. 1985). Psychiatrists or other mental health workers screen prospective candidates for IVF (Greenfield and Haseltine 1986), evaluate women who wish to be surrogate mothers (Franks 1981), provide marital counseling to couples whose infertility is causing discord (Menning 1982), and give support to couples who are grieving after IVF has failed (Rosenfield and Mitchell 1979). Psychiatrists help develop policies or guidelines about who should be accepted as a patient in a clinic and which therapies should be offered.

Given the rapid development of IVF clinics and the integral role of psychiatrists in these clinics, several areas of ethical concern relevant to psychiatrists are likely to arise. First is the problem of divided loyalty, both in regard to conflicts between particular individuals and also in regard to conflicts between individual well-being and institutional or social policy. Second, as familiarity with the new reproductive technologies increases, questions will arise about the limits of acceptable indications for these therapies. Finally, there will be ethical problems in research on the new reproductive therapies, some of which will have direct psychological implications.

Divided Loyalties

Divided loyalties often complicate psychiatric therapy. A psychiatrist, for example, may feel the need to breach patient confidentiality to protect a third party from harm. Analogous conflicts may arise in situations generated by the new reproductive technologies. If a psychiatrist is asked to evaluate potential candidates for IVF or surrogate motherhood, the psychiatrist's ethical obligations to an individual who may benefit from participation in the program may conflict with obligations to screen out unacceptable or deviant patients. The patient's best interest might conflict with the interests of the clinic, of the potential children, or of society.

Is the psychiatrist obligated to weigh the emotional health of the prospective parents against the best interests of the potential children? If so, the psychiatrist will face tremendous difficulty. Little is known of the outcomes for children conceived by the new reproductive technologies. Studies indicate that there are few short-term problems (Mushin et al. 1986; Sokoloff 1987), but some fear that the experience of these children will mirror that of adoptive children, who have a small but consistent increase in psychiatric problems. Comparisons are difficult, however, both because adoptive children comprise a very heterogeneous population and because the circumstances of adoption may predispose to psychiatric problems (Brinich and Brinich 1982).

Infertility treatment centers may use specific but somewhat arbitrary definitions of infertility; they may not accept patients over a certain age; they may require that patients be heterosexual and married. These criteria may prohibit some people access to IVF. A psychiatrist who is asked to assess or counsel such "deviant" patients must confront questions about whether it is acceptable to perpetuate standards that reflect social bias, rather than medical facts (Somerville 1982). After all, if a fertile woman wants a child, she may have one, even if she is unable to care for the child. Should infertile women be denied similar options? Psychiatrists who view reproductive freedom as an absolute right will have difficulty working in systems that have eligibility criteria based on social norms of parental acceptability.

Psychiatrists who weigh the best interest of the child above the desires of the parents will enter the ethical thicket of maternal-fetal conflicts. In obstetrics, when the interests of the mother and the interests of the fetus diverge, obstetricians must decide when a potential harm to the infant outweighs the best interest or legal rights of the mother. In the last decade, physicians have been increasingly willing to act to protect infants, even when doing so causes increased risk of harm to the mother (Rhoden 1987). Court-ordered cesarian sections have been performed in many states, and half of the directors of training programs in perinatal medicine feel that such interventions may sometimes be appropriate (Kolder et al. 1987). These cases are not quite analogous to the maternal-fetal conflicts that may arise when a woman who appears unfit to be a mother wants a child. Nevertheless, the interests of an unborn or even unconceived child, or society's interest in protecting that potential child, might, in some cases, outweigh the interests of the mother.

Particular problems may arise in surrogacy contracts. The psychiatrist may be asked to screen surrogate mother candidates to determine which women will most easily relinquish children (Parker 1983). During the pregnancy, the surrogate mother may change her mind about giving up the child. The psychiatrist may have to decide whether to "help" a patient give up her own child, against her will, to fulfill the terms of the contract or satisfy the needs of the contracting parents, or whether to support the surrogate in challenging the contract that she signed.

Another more unusual conflict of interest may arise in multiple gestations. A report by Berkowitz et al. (1988) discussed selective feticide in pregnancies involving three or more fetuses. In these cases, physicians may reduce the number of viable fetuses to give the remaining fetuses a better chance of intact survival. These techniques, like other fetal interventions, including fetal surgery, pose some risk to the mother. Choosing not to undergo the procedure also has some risks. Informed consent for such procedures should include some discussion of the psychological sequelae, as well as the likely medical outcomes.

Medical Versus Social Indications for the New Reproductive Therapies

Most of the new reproductive technologies are used only to treat infertility. As they become more widely used, the indications for their use may change. Psychiatrists may be called to counsel parents with a genetic disease (e.g., Huntington's chorea, sickle-cell disease, cystic fibrosis) to help them decide whether the risk of disease is so great that they would be willing to forgo natural reproduction. Marital stress may result if one partner prefers a natural pregnancy and the other prefers an alternative reproductive strategy.

Some individuals or couples without known genetic diseases may prefer to use an alternative reproductive strategy to choose the sex of their baby or to try to control for other characteristics (e.g., intelligence or appearance). In these cases, the ethical conflict may be between individual perceptions of the best interests of an unborn child and societal norms of behavior. A psychiatrist may be consulted to determine the motivation or competence of potential parents. Such competency decisions, when the adults have no psychiatric problems, should be recognized as attempts to mask ethical dilemmas as psychiatric problems (Perl and Shelp 1982).

These issues arise in other areas of medicine in which the goal of therapy is not to prolong life or improve health (narrowly conceived) but to augment certain functions or characteristics in already healthy people. These areas include cosmetic surgery, but also include medical therapies such as growth hormone for height augmentation, minoxidil for baldness, methylphenidate for attention-deficit hyperactivity disorder, or estrogen for the symptoms of menopause. In the future, gene therapy may offer therapies that supplement or augment natural function. These therapies are highly desirable, usually expensive, and only tangentially related to health or disease. Whether they are distributed on the basis of ability to pay or are covered by third-party payers may depend on the input of psychiatrists in determining how debilitating the social stigmatization or psychological stress associated with these conditions might be. As the indications for the new reproductive therapies broaden, psychiatrists may have to make similar determinations about various indications for various reproductive techniques.

Research Issues

The ethical issues in research derive from the conflict between a desire to provide a treatment that has a known but low success rate, and the desire to improve the treatment, even though improvements might be achieved only at some price to today's patients. This conflict is exacerbated by the fact that the treatment is elective and that most candidates for the new reproductive therapies are highly motivated people who desperately want to get pregnant.

Research into the psychiatric aspects of infertility is urgently needed. Many of the questions that need to be addressed have ethical components. For example, some investigators believe that the known neuroendocrine effects of depression may decrease fertility (Kemeter et al. 1985) and suggest that women whose infertility is secondary to psychopathology may respond less well to exogenous hormonal stimulation (Kemeter 1984). This is a controversial area of research, because infertility has only recently been classified as a medical rather than a psychological problem. Attempts to trace the links between emotions and physiology more accurately may undercut purely biochemical understandings of infertility that predominate today and may suggest that, for some women, psychotherapy may be more appropriate than IVF.

A second area of research that may have ethical implications has to do with the psychological evaluation and screening of candidates for alternative reproductive technologies. Most couples who present to infertility treatment centers are highly motivated. Few would participate in a study if they were informed that the results may disqualify them from treatment. In one study, the investigators felt that it was necessary to make clear to the patients evaluated that the results of the study would not affect their acceptance into or rejection from the program (Greenfield and Haseltine 1986). Nevertheless, the investigators worried that patients might lie out of fear that their answers might disqualify them.

Another controversial area of research will focus on the effects of alternative reproductive techniques on children. Will these children resemble adoptive children, who have a predictable increase in psychopathology? Will any new problems arise in this "experimental" population? At what point in the development of the new therapies will it be fair to say, on the basis of the outcomes for children, that they are no longer "experimental"?

Conclusions and Clinical Suggestions

Medical success in the new reproductive therapies has focused attention on a second generation of ethical questions. These do not address the absolute right or wrong of the new technologies; instead, they analyze how physicians and society should accommodate the new technologies. They are questions that must be answered in the realms of public policy, law, or economics, rather than theology or metaphysics. Two extreme views characterize the spectrum of possible responses to these issues, with a range of variations in between (Walters 1987).

The first school of thought is oriented toward individual liberties. In this school, no societal oversight of these technologies is necessary, and no societal funding for research on or dissemination of the new technologies is required. The second school of thought is oriented primarily to concerns of social welfare. It sanctions paternalistic conceptions in which physicians would act to maximize societal good, even if it meant denying individual liberties. According to this school, it would be appropriate to screen prospective parents and establish criteria for the acceptability of patients before they can avail themselves of the new reproductive technologies.

It is unlikely that, in this country, with its pluralism and its decentralized health system, that any one view will prevail as a national policy. Compromises will inevitably be reached, with room for variations in responses at the individual and institutional levels. Because of this, it is likely that many people who work in institutions that are developing programs in reproductive technology will have to confront these issues without being able to rely on national policies.

Physicians who must confront these questions should do so with cognizance of the most current scientific facts, but also with some recognition of the ancient ethical norms of medicine (Kass 1985). These ethical norms suggest certain principles that should be kept in mind by physicians in all aspects of practice, but especially in areas that involve innovative therapies.

First, the physician's primary responsibility is always to his or her individual patient. Conflicts of interest should be resolved by acting in the patient's best interest. If conflicts are unavoidable or institutionalized, the patient should be informed about them through the process of informed consent.

Second, physicians must distinguish therapies that prevent or treat diseases that cause pain, suffering, or mortality from treatments that primarily supplement, augment, or adjust a biological state that has no ill effects on health. The ethical obligation to provide the former treatments to all who need them is strong; there is no obligation to provide the latter type of treatment. Treatment of documented infertility would fall in the first category; genetic manipulation to improve appearance or the use of surrogate mothers to avoid the inconvenience of pregnancy would fall in the second category.

Finally, medical research to determine the risks and benefits of innovative therapies is essential. Patients have the right to know what is known and unknown about the risks of any procedure. They are, of course, under no obligation to participate in research. They also have no entitlement to an innovative or experimental technique, as they might for a standard therapy. Standards for determining when a therapy is no longer experimental should be especially rigorous when the therapy involves fetuses or small children. Parental consent, even when based on complete information, is not sufficient to justify research that may have risks to a child. Accordingly, research on the outcomes of new reproductive technologies from the perspective of the children produced is essential.

References

Berger D: Infertility: a psychiatrist's perspective. Can J Psychiatry 25:553–558, 1980

Berkowitz RL, Lynch L, Chitkara U, et al: Selective reduction of multifetal pregnancies in the first trimester. N Engl J Med 318:1043–1047, 1988

Brinich PM, Brinich EB: Adoption and adaptation. J Nerv Ment Dis 170:489–493, 1982

DeVries WC: The physician, the media, and the 'spectacular' case. JAMA 259:886–890, 1988

Edwards RG: The scientific basis of ethics. Ann NY Acad Sci 442:564–570, 1985

Edwards RG, Bavister BD, Steptoe PC: Early stages of fertilization in vitro in human oocytes matured in vitro. Nature 221:632–635, 1969

Edwards RG, Steptoe PC, Purdy JM: Fertilization and cleavage in vitro of preovulatory human oocyte. Nature 227:1307–1309, 1970

Franks DD: Psychiatric evaluation of women in a surrogate mother program. Am J Psychiatry 138:1378–1379, 1981

Freeman EW, Boxer AS, Rickles K, et al: Psychological evaluation and support in a program of in vitro fertilization and embryo transfer. Fertil Steril 43:48, 1985

Greenfield D, Haseltine F: Candidate selection and psychosocial considerations of in vitro fertilization procedures. Clin Obstet Gynecol 29:119–126, 1986

Henahan JF: Fertilization, embryo transfer procedures raise many questions. JAMA 252:877–882, 1984

Kass LR: Babies by means of in vitro fertilization: unethical experiments on the unborn? N Engl J Med 285:1174–1179, 1971

Kass L: The ends of medicine and the pursuit of health, in Toward a More Natural Science. New York, Free Press, 1985, pp 157–186

Kemeter P: Idiopathic infertility and IVF-ET (abstract). Experientia 40:233, 1984

Kemeter P, Eder A, Springer-Krenser M: Psychosocial testing and pre-treatment of women for in vitro fertilization. Ann NY Acad Sci 442:523–532, 1985

Kolder VEB, Gallagher J, Parsons MT: Court ordered obstetrical interventions. N Engl J Med 316:1192–1196, 1987

Menning BE: The emotional needs of infertile couples. Fertil Steril 37:137, 1982

Mushin DN, Barreeda-Hanson MC, Spensley JC: In vitro fertilization children: early psychosocial development. J In Vitro Fert Embryo Transfer 3:247–252, 1986

NC Documentary Service: Instruction on Respect for Human Life in Its Origin and on the Dignity of Procreation. Origins, NC Documentary Service. Rome, Vatican Printing Office, March 19, 1987; 16:698–711

Parker PJ: Motivation of surrogate mothers: initial findings. Am J Psychiatry 140:117–118, 1983

Perl M, Shelp EE: Psychiatric consultation masking moral dilemmas in medicine. N Engl J Med 307:618–621, 1982

Raymond CA: In vitro fertilization enters stormy adolescence as experts debate the odds. JAMA 259:464–469, 1988

Rhoden NK: Caesareans and samaritans. Law, Medicine and Health Care 15:118–126, 1987

Rosenfield D, Mitchell E: Treating the emotional aspects of infertility: counseling services in an infertility clinic. Am J Obstet Gynecol 135:177, 1979

Sokoloff BZ: Alternative methods of reproduction: effects on the child. Clin Pediatr (Phila) 26:11–17, 1987

Somerville MA: Birth technology, parenting and deviance. Int J Law Psychiatry 5:123–153, 1982

Steptoe P: Historical aspects of the ethics of in vitro fertilization. Ann NY Acad Sci 442:573–576, 1985

Steptoe PC, Edwards RG: The research of today and the ethics of tomorrow. Br Med J 3:342–343, 1972

Walters L: Human in vitro fertilization: a review of the ethical literature. Hastings Cent Rep 9:23, 1979

Walters L: Test-tube babies: Ethical considerations. Clin Perinatol 14:271–280, 1987

Weaver DD, Escobar LF: Twenty-four ways to have children. Am J Med Genet 26:737–740, 1987

Chapter 8

Psychological Ramifications of "Surrogate" Motherhood

Michelle Harrison, M.D.

What has been will be again,
what has been done will be done again;
there is nothing new under the sun. (Ecclesiastes 1:9)

The past 10 years have brought with them a revolution in the treatment of infertility and the technology of conception. The future promises—or maybe threatens—even more profound changes in how new human beings are planned, created, designed, screened, and distributed. Yet, with all this change before us, we remain the same human beings with the same emotions, thoughts, yearnings, and conflicts. The issues of fertility, fidelity, heritage, class, and motherhood affect us as deeply as ever. The ancient themes of Judeo-Christian culture and religion are played out over and over again, with only the centuries and the names of the individuals changed.

In the Holy Bible (1984), when Sarah urged Abraham to sleep with her maidservant Hagar, and thus produce an heir, all did not go smoothly. On conception, Hagar came to despise Sarah. Sarah mistreated Hagar, who ran away. Only by the intervention of the angel of God did Hagar return to bear Abraham his son Ishmael. Sarah eventually conceived, but on the weaning of her son Isaac, she commanded that Abraham banish Hagar and Ishmael.

Millenia later, Mary Beth Whitehead gave birth to a child she was to have given to William Stern, the baby's father. All did not go well, and the case of Baby M subsequently resulted in highly polarized views of surrogacy, technology, motherhood, the legal system, and psychiatry. The case of Mary Beth Whitehead, Elizabeth Stern, Bill Stern, and Sara/Melissa

Whitehead/Stern caught the imagination, fantasies, and judgment of the world. There were few people who failed to hold or express strong and highly invested opinions in that case.

No new reproductive technology was used, but the case seems to have symbolized both the hopes and fears of a population regarding the future composition of families and the production of children. Although Baby M was not about donor eggs or embryo transfer, the proximity of issues and questions raised contributed to its highly charged atmosphere.

The Baby M case is simple compared with what lies ahead. While many invoked the "Wisdom of Solomon," in fact there was never any question as to who the mother of the child was. Solomon was faced with not knowing which of two women had given birth to the baby in question. In Baby M a contract existed, one that was eventually ruled void and illegal by the New Jersey Supreme Court, but there never was doubt as to either whose "egg" contributed to the child or in whose body she had gestated. As to who "should" be the mother, that took on all the social, class, and professional biases inherent in any custody struggle played out in the public arena. Some identified with the child, some with the "infertile couple," and some with the mother.

But the case was also full of "what ifs." What if the egg had belonged to Betsy Stern? What if the egg had belonged to yet another woman, but had been gestated with the intent of giving the child to the Sterns? What if the sperm had been someone else's? What if there had been no money exchange? What if the baby had died in utero? What if she had been born deformed? What if Mary Beth Whitehead had chosen to abort? What if the Sterns had requested that she abort? What if she died? What if Bill Stern died?

We are poised on the brink of new technologies that will separate human reproduction as we have known it from the creation of new humans. The potential chaos that looms before us today probably leaves us as bewildered as our forbearers who had not yet connected coitus and genes with pregnancy and childbirth.

As we try to create order and understanding of what lies ahead, it is important to see what we can learn from those individuals whose lives have already been affected by new reproductive arrangements.

Franks (1981) reported on 10 women accepted into a surrogacy program who had been administered the Minnesota Multiphasic Personality Inventory. He found no psychopathology in 9. The other was hypomanic. Individual profiles of the women showed high femininity and social extroversion scores. Their average age was 26 years. Each had one to three living children. Nine women had been married at least once, 4 were divorced, and 1 was single. Women reported their reasons for wanting to be surrogate mothers as being a history of positive experiences with pregnancy and labor, love for their own children, the desire to share this love, and a need for financial remuneration.

Parker (1983) reported on 125 of 225 women he had interviewed as part of their applications to become surrogate mothers. Their mean age was 25; 56% were married, 20% divorced, and the rest single. Of the women, 91% had one previous pregnancy; 81% had at least one previous live birth, with the average being 1.7. There was a history of previous pregnancy loss in 35%.

Parker (1983) described the motivation of women for surrogacy as related to a need for money, enjoyment of pregnancy, a wish to give "the gift of a baby to a parent who needed a child," and a belief, which he says was often unconscious, that this experience would help the women resolve feelings about past pregnancy loss, either through abortion or relinquishment of a child. These findings are similar to Franks's (1981), with the exception of the relevance of past pregnancies (not presented by Franks). Beyond the demographics, it is important to understand on a more individual basis some of what motivates these women to act as "surrogates."

A Need to Feel Special

Women appear to enter into these agreements with almost an innocence, or fairy-tale quality. Chesler (1988) described an "almost stubborn naivete exhibited by these women." They are giving "the gift of life" (M.B. Whitehead, unpublished, 1985) to someone who cannot have a baby, and part of their reward is a sense of specialness, a sense of importance. Some do it anonymously—that is, without knowing the sperm donor/couple before they become pregnant. Elizabeth Kane (1988), the first paid commercial surrogate mother in the United States, wrote of feeling "suffocated" by the desperation of a sister, a brother, and two cousins who had been unable to have children and feeling "guilty about her own fertility." Then, after reading a newspaper advertisement, she said, "Suddenly a feeling swept over me—a knowledge that I would have a child for this couple in Kentucky" (p. 14). When her husband protested and asked who these people were, she replied, "I don't know. They just need a baby" (p. 16).

The sense of specialness has been reinforced if not created by the advertising of the surrogacy programs and by the media attention to surrogacy as a solution to the pain of infertility. Brodsky (1988) reported that "there may be unrealistic psychological needs to be special, loved, or appreciated." Some of these women seem to have felt driven to have and to be able to give away these babies. For some, surrogacy may have seemed to offer a moment of glory, a chance at the stars, of meaning beyond one's own life—their own seat on the Challenger Shuttle.

The Ability to Perceive the Baby as "Not Mine"

Reality often becomes defined by the language we use. In most situations, a woman who gives birth, whatever she does afterward, is a mother. To be a surrogate is to be a substitute. The term *surrogate mother* is used to imply that the pregnant woman (mother) is substituting for the "real" mother, the wife of the father. In Baby M, the press and often the courts referred to Mary Beth Whitehead as the surrogate mother, and Bill Stern as the "natural" father. It was not until the oral arguments before the New Jersey Supreme Court that the judicial system referred to Mary Beth Whitehead as the mother or natural mother, to Bill Stern alternately as the sperm donor or natural father, and to Betsy Stern as the stepmother. Interestingly, but not surprising, the change in language coincided with a reversal of the findings and decision of the lower court regarding parental rights and visitation. The question of language will become even more critical as we separate egg donation from gestation.

Throughout most of these women's pregnancies (with this aspect shifting for some women as they approach birth), the fetus is perceived as belonging to the "other woman." The pregnant woman tells herself, and has tremendous support for the belief, that this is not her baby. The medical health care team reinforce that she is carrying someone else's baby. Cohen and Friend (1987) quoted Bill Handel, an attorney who arranges surrogate agreements, as saying that the surrogate "must absolutely understand and believe the child she is carrying is not hers, but instead belongs to the couple from the moment of insemination" (p. 288). Parker (1983) described women as saying, "I'd be nest watching," or most definitively, "It would be their baby, not mine." He said the women tended to deny their attachment to the baby, often seeing themselves as incubators or as taking care of the other woman's baby.

The woman tells her other children that the baby is not hers, that it belongs to the other couple. The basis for that belief becomes the contractual arrangement and the sperm donor/father's contribution. She does not appear to say to herself, "I am giving up my baby." Dr. Lee Salk's description of Mary Beth Whitehead as a "surrogate uterus" reinforced that perception. This perception on the part of the women may also be supported by the psychiatric evaluations required for entry into such programs. Basically all surrogacy programs utilize some form of screening. One may screen for informed consent only. Another may try to assess the woman's ability to relinquish a child and may act as more or less of an advisor or even a "gatekeeper." In any event, a woman entering the program at some point must be in some way "cleared" to continue. Such clearance must add to her sense that in some way what she is doing makes sense and that her participation has been endorsed by the mental health community.

Many surrogacy contracts include a provision that the surrogate mother not form any emotional attachment to the child. Despite this proviso, Nancy Reame (1984) reported that six of eight women reported that they had come to love the baby by the ninth gestational month. For the women who are unsuccessful surrogates, *it is the fantasy that the baby is not theirs* that breaks down, and it happens at various times. I will describe three well-known cases and how that breakdown occurred at different times.

Case 1. Alejandra Munoz is a Mexican woman brought illegally across the border to be a surrogate mother for a cousin in California. She was 19 years old and had a child. She had completed fourth grade but could not read. She believed that she was coming to the United States to be inseminated by her cousin's husband and then to donate the embryo to her cousin. Because she knew of similar procedures with cattle, she believed this is what would occur. Several weeks after the insemination she realized that she was actually going to have a baby. She considered an abortion, but because of her religion and family pressure, agreed to carry to term. She felt the baby to be hers and did not intend to relinquish the child. The rest of this story is less relevant in terms of dynamics, but she has been embroiled in a lengthy and nasty custody battle. She has had visitation with her daughter throughout this time.

Case 2. Mary Beth Whitehead believed she was carrying Betsy and Bill Stern's baby for most of the pregnancy. In the final month, she began to have some thoughts about its being "her" baby. Some of this occurred around differences between the two women that became apparent at that time. For Mary Beth, the prospect of Betsy's returning to work immediately conflicted with her own beliefs about mothers staying home with their children. For awhile they even talked about Mary Beth being the babysitter while Betsy worked. It was in the birth process that Mary Beth experienced the baby as hers. She described the pain of labor, and the fact that the baby came out looking just like her other children, as leading to her realization that the child was her own. The rest of that case is well known.

Case 3. Elizabeth Kane delivered her child in November 1980 after traveling the country promoting surrogacy on major television shows. Kane (1988) wrote: "For months following the birth I was euphoric. I would get high just remembering the look on Adam's and Margo's faces as they held their son in the delivery room" (p. 276). By the time he was 8 months old, she was "unable to push away the thought of him. . . . and I began to acknowledge the dull aching in the middle of my chest" (p. 276). She apparently lapsed into a severe depression. "The depression soon grew into fantasies of my death. I had assured myself [that] Kent and the children, as well as Margo and Adam would be better off without me. I was a blight that needed to be removed" (p. 277). Part of her conflict throughout that time related to her wish not to be seen as a surrogacy failure.

Kane's depression eventually lifted, but it was not until 1986 when she saw a story about Mary Beth Whitehead in *People Weekly* that she began to speak publicly about the emotional aftermath for her and her family. "Tears streaming down my face, I admitted to the press that I missed my son, that

I had never gotten over the loss of him and that surrogate motherhood was a terrible mistake" (Kane 1988, p. 285).

These are three women reflecting three different time periods in which they shifted their perceptions regarding whose child they were carrying. For Munoz it was shortly after conception, for Whitehead it was at the time of birth, and for Kane it was in the months after her son's birth. Those surrogate mothers who remain publicly supportive of surrogacy continue to refer to themselves as carrying someone else's child.

Idealization of the Parental Couple or Man

At the same time the women were carrying the "other woman's" baby, they were also carrying (more realistically) the other man's baby. They tended to idealize the couple, often on the basis of minimal or no information. Kane (1988) reported: "I knew they would be good parents. Adam would be a perfect father." As for Adam's wife, "I couldn't have handpicked a better woman . . . attractive and sensitive. . . . She would put her own ambitions aside to raise my son" (p. 218). Franks (1981) reported that "these women felt assured that the background and characteristics of the family who would be rearing the child were good" (p. 379). Parker (1984) reported that "they tended to feel, 'they will be good loving parents and I like them very much' " (p. 8).

In addition to idealization, there is often an attachment to the man or to the couple. There can also be a sense of competition between the surrogate mother and the wife. It is not uncommon for the families to become close during the pregnancy, an attempt at becoming one big happy family. Not surprising, the prospective parental couple tends to be more open, or even welcoming of the relationship with the surrogate mother and her family, before the birth than after. Chesler (1988) reported similar findings among the women she interviewed. Parker (1984) reported that some surrogates "felt most of their sadness in connection with the loss of the relationship with the couple rather than the loss of the baby" (p. 11). He added that "they often felt angry and unhappy about the enforced exile from the parental couple and their new child" (p. 12). In cases in which the relationship with the sperm donor/father has become sexualized, the woman experiences both the loss of the baby and the loss of that relationship. The woman may also identify with her baby and thus live vicariously through her child's being reared by the idealized parental couple.

Pregnancy Loss or Relinquishment

In Parker's (1983) sample, 26% had had a previous abortion and 9% had relinquished a child for adoption. He described one woman who felt that she was giving a child to a couple instead of "killing a baby." She had had a previous abortion. Parker (1984) felt that relinquishing a baby helped the woman deal with unresolved voluntary losses. Brodsky (1988) described this as psychological compensation for previous losses or failures—abortions, lack of self-esteem, or goals in life. One might question, however, especially in the absence of a therapeutic context, whether giving away a baby would result in a woman's feeling better about having lost one before. Nevertheless, this is one of the benefits of surrogacy touted in the media and by the industry. Parker (1984) reported that some surrogate mothers expressed a wish to have a "replacement child" after relinquishing the surrogacy child. Mary Beth Whitehead became pregnant within months of Judge Sorkow's decision to terminate her parental rights to her child.

Need for Financial Remuneration

Although it is generally agreed that without the money there would be far fewer volunteers for surrogacy, for many of these women the money may not be the prime motivation. That may not be true in the future, both as the novelty diminishes and as the surrogacy industry tries to widen its pool of women, because some of the sense of "specialness" may be lost. Parker (1984) reported that the concept of "fee for service" may result in less anxiety and guilt than payment for termination of parental rights. Franks (1981) described one motivational factor as being "a need for the financial remuneration to stabilize their personal lives and to provide for their *own* [emphasis added] children's needs" (p. 1379). Parker (1983) reported that 89% of the women felt a fee was necessary, but was not a sufficient reason itself. Brodsky (1988) likewise reported that financial compensation is a motivational factor for surrogate mothers. Surrogacy has so far attracted women from a wide economic range. Presumably, for those women on welfare or who are economically marginal, the fee is of more importance than for those more economically comfortable. However, it is also possible that for women under severe economic conditions, the chance at "specialness" may be equally or even more enticing.

Women With Children

While not universally true, most programs will not accept a woman unless she already has children. Although there has been much speculation about the effects on the surrogacy children, their half siblings have been ignored. There has been little consideration of their needs and vulnerability and there has been no follow-up. Pannor (unpublished, 1986) said of the siblings that surrogacy "can only cause them to wonder what kind of values exist in their family. Should the family be in economic straits in the future, the children may naturally wonder if they could be the next to be sacrificed." Brodsky

(1988) said that the "relationship between the surrogate and her existing children and spouse might be at risk."

These children may be at very high risk, even more so than the surrogacy children themselves. Most of the siblings have been old enough to know of their mother's pregnancy. Told that the baby about to be born is not really a sibling, they are confronted with a discordance between their own perceptions and what they are being told. In addition, they do not share in the sense of "specialness" of their mothers, nor have they had any control over the process. Some of the older siblings have experienced shame and embarrassment at their mothers' pregnancies. Steadman and McCloskey (1987) wrote: "Increased abandonment anxiety is a distinct possibility in the children of surrogate families who see their parents willingly giving away children after birth" (p. 547). These authors further reminded us of the serious depressive reactions in children who experience sibling loss through death, family breakdown, and child protection litigation.

After the birth, many of these mothers are dealing with sadness and anger over the loss of the child and maybe of the relationship with the couple as well (Parker 1984). Reame (1987) reported that 50% may experience moderate symptoms of perinatal loss. It would be difficult in the months following the birth for these women to address the needs and reactions of their other children adequately. If relinquishment requires a detachment from the child in utero, it may be impossible for them to understand the responses of siblings who may have formed an attachment to their sibling-to-be. Siblings may be left with confusion, guilt, and fear of their own abandonment. They may also simply experience the loss of a sibling who, despite what they had been told, they expected to know as a part of their family.

Elizabeth Kane (1988) wrote of the emotional impact of giving away a sibling on her other three children. Each has apparently suffered in relation to that loss, their reactions including sadness, anger, shame, withdrawal, and fearfulness. At times, the children as well as their mothers must grieve the loss of the other family. Often there has been almost a blending of families during the pregnancy. Hard as it is to believe today, the Whiteheads and Sterns were close during the pregnancy. The Sterns came to watch the older children play soccer. Ten-year-old Tuesday Whitehead stayed overnight at the Sterns' home and went to the Macy's Day Parade in New York. There are many other similar stories of the families joined in their mutual fantasy of being one big happy family. Chesler (1988) described one woman telling her son that the baby would be like a cousin to him, that he "would always be able to see it, play with it, grow up knowing the baby" (p. 58).

The children have not always been passive observers, but rather active participants. Tuesday Whitehead begged the Sterns to call off the police who had handcuffed her mother and taken her from the house. Months later she used a hairbrush to try to fight off the detectives who seized the baby in Florida. Back in New Jersey, Tuesday insisted that her sister's crib remain in her room. While the media, the experts, and courts may have accused her mother of using her, of prolonging the trauma by not disposing of the empty crib, such a position does not do justice to the feelings of the siblings of the children who are being given away. In a time of war, this 10-year-old's acts would have been seen as heroic, and to this child, the actions of the trusted adults in her life, both her parents and the Sterns, had created a battleground. Like the child who called out "The Emperor has no clothes!" these siblings are not as vulnerable to, nor invested in, the belief that the baby inside "mommy's tummy" is no relation of theirs.

I have not addressed the issue of the surrogate children themselves. We can speculate what the effects on them will be, and it will probably be some combination of reactions to adoption and stepparenting. Whether they will feel more wanted or less wanted because of their special origins will obviously vary and may also be different at different stages in their lives. However, since the oldest child is only 8 years of age, and since they are generally not available for study, those answers will be slow in coming. Likewise, little is known about the fathers and their wives. Information in the literature has come through those involved in the private industry of surrogacy. It is a buyer's market in which women (and their children) are screened and catalogued while the parental couple chooses. Since the father already has a claim on the child, the usual safeguards of adoption are not required.

Although legislators and the courts have addressed mainly commercial surrogacy—that is, where money is exchanged and third parties are involved—from a psychological viewpoint, the potential for interpersonal difficulties is as great when surrogacy occurs within a family or between friends. The Munoz case has torn that family apart. Another case involving sisters is being battled across a continent. Another case of sisters has resulted in a baby with acquired immunodeficiency syndrome (AIDS) who remains hospitalized because neither woman wants him (Frederick et al. 1987). A 10-year friendship between two women ended after one became a surrogate for the other. Although noncommercial in-family or between-friends surrogacy may at times meet the needs of everyone concerned, we have to remember that coercion within families can be as strong as any monetary inducement. When it does not work out, the family members still must relate to each other over time.

The Role of the Psychiatrist

The Bible is unclear as to whether Abraham and Sarah consulted with anyone before approaching Hagar to bear Abraham a child. Likewise, it seems doubtful that Hagar had benefit of psychological consultation before agreeing to conceive a child. Less is known about Ishmael. Whether the Bible represents history or metaphor, its stories and themes continue to have meaning for us. In the 20th century we often turn to medicine and to psychiatry in our attempt to create order and find meaning in our lives. Today, Abraham and Sarah might have consulted with a psychiatrist before deciding to embark on surrogacy. Hagar would probably have been required to have a psychological examination before being accepted as a surrogate mother. Ishmael would have been studied carefully, his growth and development watched to see the effect of being a child of a surrogate. When trouble arose, the courts would have called in mental health experts to help decide the fate of Ishmael and Hagar. Finally, years later, Isaac would have appeared on "The Phil Donahue Show" in his search for his lost brother Ishmael!

The major roles of the psychiatrist in surrogate motherhood are in the decision-making process and as experts in the courts.

Gatekeeper

The psychiatrist may have the power to accept or refuse applicants into a surrogacy program or agreement. This power and role may be limited to the surrogate mother applicant or might include the contracting man or couple. Private programs have tended to screen the mothers but not the contracting man or couple. University-based programs, especially ones that are beginning to include embryo transfer and egg donation, may screen all parties. It is not clear what criteria are used.

It is important to know why a psychiatrist is being used for this purpose. What is the real purpose of the psychiatrist's role? Is the program genuinely worried about the participants? Is the program worried about a lawsuit? Is the program using psychiatric screening to legitimize the process? Is it for public relations?

There are already well-developed criteria used for adoption home studies. However, often individuals and couples turning to surrogacy are unable to meet the criteria of various state agencies regarding adoption. Others are offended at having to be "screened" to adopt a child. Many of the couples are ones in which the woman has already had children by another man, but is now older and either voluntarily or involuntarily infertile. Therefore, the population seeking surrogate services will have to be screened by some other criteria. By definition, they will not be the traditional ones.

Creating criteria for the surrogate mothers is equally difficult. What makes a good or satisfied surrogate mother? What is needed to perceive a child in utero as "not mine?" We still know little of these women's backgrounds. Chesler (1988) alluded to frequent histories of sexual abuse among these women. Parker (1983) and Brodsky (1988) referred to previous pregnancy loss. Whether such histories should be criteria of inclusion or exclusion and what effect repeated loss will have are still unknown.

The psychiatrist who acts as gatekeeper must be able to explain accepting as well as rejecting applicants. Does acceptance of contracting couples or individuals indicate that they will be good parents? That they are "healthy"? That they have a good relationship? That they have a "right" to a child by these means? Does rejection imply the opposites of the above? As for the surrogate mother, does acceptance imply that she "should" go ahead or will be able to go ahead with the surrogacy arrangement? Does it imply endorsement? In the years before *Roe v. Wade*, many states required psychiatric examination before a woman could have a therapeutic abortion. Such requirements do not exist at present. In that situation a woman had to convince a psychiatrist that she would be psychologically unhealthy if she had to carry a pregnancy to term. Physicians learned how to "pass" women, and women learned how to answer questions so as to have the requested abortion. The potential exists for psychiatrists to function in a similar role in new reproductive technologies.

Advisor to the Woman Considering Surrogacy

The psychiatrist may be consulted by any of the parties requesting assistance in the decision. Given how little we know at present about the consequences of surrogacy, our most important role may be to help people anticipate what some of their responses and reactions might be. For purposes of this chapter, only noncommercial surrogacy will be addressed. The question of legality remains in flux, both in the United States and internationally. In addition, there is an entirely different set of ethical questions to be raised when money is transferred in exchange for a child.

For the woman considering surrogacy, several areas should be addressed.

Motivation. What is the primary inner need that she is attempting to meet? Is she doing this for strangers, relatives, or friends? Is she under duress from others? If the motivation is related to meaning in her life, what other options might she have? How does she expect to feel? Does she want a child herself? Does she feel guilty about having children herself when the others do not? Does she have other guilts that may seem to be assuaged by giving a child to someone else? Is she motivated by religious beliefs? Abraham later proved his loyalty to God by offering to sacrifice his son. Christ was God's sacrifice to save the world.

Previous childbearing loss. Has she experienced losses? How does she see this experience in relation to previous losses? How has she resolved feelings and/or conflicts about previous losses? Is she seeking punishment or absolution or some of each?

Family support. What are the feelings of the woman's spouse? Her mother? Her father? Has she discussed her plans with them? Will they feel they are grandparents, and thus feel the loss of a grandchild? Does the woman have other children? The special issues of siblings have been addressed earlier. How has or will she prepare them or support them through their loss of a sibling?

Perception of the father or couple.   How does she view the father or couple? Has she idealized them? How does she imagine their relationship to be in the future? Is she realistic? What are her own feelings about family or belonging? Does she expect them to feel grateful? How grateful?

Perception of the child.   Will she perceive the child as hers or as the father's? Obviously this is the most difficult question to answer, but it may be one of the most important ones. Anticipating *a* baby is different from seeing one's own baby. It is important for a woman contemplating surrogacy to find ways of perceiving the child as real to try to anticipate her reactions. She should be encouraged to think about her own style of mothering, and then how it would feel to have her child raised in another style. Mundane as it might seem, people may have very strong reactions to such issues as whether to use a pacifier, whether the baby will be fed on a schedule or on demand, when to wean, whether the baby will sleep alone or in the parental bed. When such questions are addressed, the child-to-be is less a concept and more an individual, and a woman's ability to anticipate her reactions may be more accurate.

Advisor to the Couple Considering Surrogacy

The couple considering surrogacy have a different set of questions to answer.

Motivations.   Why are they choosing surrogacy? If the woman is infertile, to what extent has she resolved her feelings? To what extent has the man resolved his feelings about his wife's infertility? Do they both want the child? Does either of them already have children from other relationships or marriages? Do they have adopted children? How does the woman feel about her husband's ability to father a child? Does she anticipate the surrogacy child as making her feel more or less conflicted about her infertility? What do they anticipate to be an advantage of genetic linkage? What are their beliefs as to what traits are inherited? How do they anticipate that a child of surrogacy will or will not be different from an adopted child?

Relationship with the mother.   What do they anticipate to be the future relationship? Here it is probably important to make the woman real—as important as it is for the mother to make the child real. For the couple, especially for the woman, the possibility of the mother's remaining in the child's life is one that must be anticipated. When surrogacy takes place within a family, this is inevitable. For the woman there is the question of jealousy of the relationship between her husband and the mother. The romanticizing of the relationship between the father and the mother is a possibility. Again, there is a difference between *a* woman who will relinquish her child and the child's mother. The question of gratitude is as important for the couple as for the mother. How grateful will they feel, and then how will they feel about that gratitude? Will that ultimately endear the woman to them, or will it become resentment?

Family and others.   What are the feelings of parents and other relatives? If there are other children in the family, either children of one of the partners or adopted children, what are their feelings? What do they perceive as the motivation of their parents?

The children of surrogacy.   What is the image of the child for the couple? What needs do they expect the child to meet? How do they perceive this child as same or different from other children? What do they anticipate to be the problems? What do they plan to say? This is probably one of the more difficult areas to anticipate and is probably ultimately of less importance at the time of initial consideration of surrogacy. Just as a woman's perception may change with the birth of a child, so do the ways in which people then parent children. The journey from initial consideration of surrogacy to the birth of the child is such a long one emotionally that there may be little similarity between how one anticipates dealing with some issues and how one eventually does so. In addition, the child may by its own personality and needs partly determine what will be said and when. However, for purposes of exploration of feelings, the topic is a useful one even in the early stages of consideration.

The Psychiatrist as Expert Witness

Expert witnesses are needed only in times of conflict. They become advisors to the court when questions seem to go beyond law per se. The courts have turned to mental health experts in contested surrogacy cases, much as they have done in routine custody cases. For the most part, the courts have directed the experts to examine the principals, ignoring the contractual aspect of the child's conception. However, despite these instructions, experts have tended to give greater attention to the father's wife and have entertained opinions regarding termination of parental rights in the absence of usual grounds (*In the Matter of Baby M* 1987). For instance, in an ordinary custody case involving a divorce or breakup of the relationship between a man and a woman, the man's new wife is not considered competitively as a mother to the child. She is part of the father's home, but she is not evaluated with regard to whether she or the child's mother should be the mother to the child. The only exceptions to this would be in situations of abuse or neglect, none of which were present in Baby M. In the case of Alejandra Munoz described earlier, the expert reports clearly compared which of the two women would make the better mother to the child. The issue is an important one because, in general, we do not assess custody cases with regard to where we can find a better mother for a child, but rather, given this child with these two parents, where do we believe the child will do best. In ordinary custody cases, we recognize that the mother will be the mother and the father will remain the father, although obviously their respective spouses and family members will play important roles in the child's life.

The added difficulty of experts is with respect to class, economic, and educational biases (Harrison 1987a). In the cases of surrogacy in which the mother is paid for the child, there is presumably an economic differential between the father and the mother. The New Jersey Supreme Court stated: "we doubt that infertile couples in the low-income bracket will find upper income surrogates" (*In the Matter of Baby M* 1988, p. 50).

Directions for Research

It is clear that research has been limited to date, and yet in its absence we remain partly in limbo. As mentioned, the participants in new reproductive technology have been relatively unavailable for study. This is a result of the circumstances under which contracts have been made, partly because of the reluctance of participants to offer themselves for further intrusion into their lives and partly because even the questions themselves are difficult to frame. Clearly the children, the mothers, the siblings, and the receiving parents all need to be understood and followed. The question of genetic linkage is as much a cultural issue as a biological one, and yet it too must be better understood. We believe we have an understanding of genes, and yet we know little about the effect of that knowledge on our lives. As the composition of families continues to shift, as it has in the past few decades, the combinations of parent, stepparents, and gestation, genetic, birth, and social parents add new challenges to our attempts to understand the nature of human relationships and our role in trying to improve the quality and nature of those lives. Some of that can occur only as we continue to explore the process and the individuals whose lives are affected or even created by the new reproductive technologies.

Social Policy

Although it is important to examine the characteristics, dynamics, and experiences of the individuals involved in surrogacy, we should not ignore the social policy issues raised. First of all, as psychiatrists, our opinions and experiences are often considered valuable if not essential in creating social policy. We are called on by courts, by legislators, and by the media. Second, our participation in cases involving surrogacy, whether as part of a program or as expert witnesses, usually places us in positions of opposition or endorsement. Likewise, our treatment of any participant of surrogacy will be influenced by our assessments of both the psychological and social policy aspects of this practice. As much as we may attempt neutrality, whether we see surrogacy as a supreme act of altruism or of exploitation will affect our judgment. Whether we see surrogate mothers as courageous pioneers in a Brave New World or lemmings heading to the sea will determine whether we help create pathways, supports, or barriers.

There are troubling questions we must ask ourselves. Do we see genetic linkage as necessity or narcissism? What is the meaning of eugenics in these new practices and new technologies? Do we see the demand for Caucasian babies as racism (Harrison 1987b), or as Steadman and McCloskey (1987) wrote, that "the couple . . . are rejecting, as they have every right to do, the option of adopting a child of different racial background, an older child, or a handicapped child" (p. 48). It is unlikely that women of means will have babies for poor women, but rather the reverse. Is that exploitation or opportunity? As we move into more technological forms of creating babies, how do we value genes and gestation, and how does that relate to our concepts of "family"? If a woman gestates the egg of another woman, is she the mother or is the egg donor the mother? Where we find ourselves on the spectrum of answers to these questions will have an impact not only on individuals we treat but also on those areas of our culture and society in which our thoughts and opinions are sought.

References

Brodsky AM: Ethical perspectives of surrogate motherhood. Paper presented at the National Conference on Birth, Death, and Law, American Bar Association, Philadelphia, PA, February 4–5, 1988

Chesler P: Sacred Bond: The Legacy of Baby M. New York, Times Books, 1988

Cohen B, Friend TL: Legal and ethical implications of surrogate mother contracts. Clin Perinatol 14:281–292, 1987

Franks DD: Psychiatric evaluation of women in a surrogate mother program. Am J Psychiatry 138:1378–1379, 1981

Frederick WR, Delapenha R, Gray G, et al: HIV testing of surrogate mothers. N Engl J Med 317:1351, 1987

Harrison M: Social construction of Mary Beth Whitehead. Gender and Society 1:300–311, 1987a

Harrison M: Women as breeders? ethical and racial issues. News for Women in Psychiatry 5:1–2, 1987b

Holy Bible, New International Version. London, Hodder and Stoughton, 1984

In the Matter of Baby M, Doc No FM25314-86E, Chan Div/Fam Pt, Bergen Co Sup Ct NJ, 1987

In the Matter of Baby M, A-39-87, NJ Sup Ct decision February 3, 1988

Kane E: Birth Mother. New York, Harcourt Brace Jovanovich, 1988

Parker PJ: Motivation of surrogate mothers: initial findings. Am J Psychiatry 140:117–118, 1983

Parker PJ: The psychology of the pregnant surrogate mother: a newly updated report of a longitudinal pilot study. Paper presented at the American Orthopsychiatric Association meeting, Toronto, April 9, 1984

Reame NE: The development of a perinatal nursing service for the surrogate mother (abstract). J Obstet Gynecol Neonatal Nurs, Jan–Feb, 1984, p 59

Reame NE: Maternal adaptation and psychologic responses to a surrogate pregnancy. Abstract presented at the American Fertility Society, September 28–30, 1987, p 37

Steadman JH, McCloskey GT: The prospect of surrogate mothering: clinical concerns. Can J Psychiatry 32:545–550, 1987

Chapter 9

Single Women Requesting Artificial Insemination by Donor

Miriam B. Rosenthal, M.D.

A rtificial insemination with donor sperm as a remedy for male infertility has been technically possible for more than 200 years (Beck 1984). It is not "high tech" but shares with the other newer reproductive technologies intense emotions, secrecy, and religious controversies—especially when it is used by unmarried women.

The first recorded artificial insemination by husband was in 1790. Dr. John Hunter was consulted by a couple because of infertility. The husband had hypospadias. Husband and wife were shown how to take a syringe, collect semen, and inject it into the vagina. It was done at home and pregnancy ensued (Corea 1979).

The first insemination with donor sperm that was recorded by an observer several years after it had happened occurred in Philadelphia in 1884. The observers had been pledged to secrecy for years. A couple sought the help of a Professor Pancoast about their infertility. The husband was azoospermic. The wife was anesthesized with chloroform in the operating room, and the "best looking medical student" was chosen for the donor. Then the semen was deposited in the uterus with a syringe. A pregnancy resulted. The husband was told, but not the wife (Corea 1979)!

In 1986 the American Fertility Society published its newest guidelines for use of donor semen for insemination (Peterson 1986). The main purpose of these guidelines was to improve donor selection, decrease the possibility of infection, improve the technology, and look at areas needing further monitoring and follow-up studies. Psychological evaluation and counseling were recommended. Indications were summarized as follows:

1. Husband's sterility due to azoospermia from any cause.
2. Husband's sterility from a vasectomy he does not wish to or cannot reverse.
3. Husband's oligospermia, or seminal fluid abnormality associated with male factor infertility.
4. Husband's genetic or hereditary disorder (Tay-Sachs, Huntington's chorea, other chromosomal abnormalities).
5. Husband's difficulty with ejaculation, secondary to trauma, surgery, or drugs, that is noncorrectable.
6. Wife's Rh negative blood type, with Rh isoimmunization and Rh positive husband.

The donor evaluation process requires screening the donor: determination of good health as confirmed by a careful history and physical examination, absence of genetic disease, and age less than 50 years.

The semen must be of sufficient volume (i.e., greater than 2 ml). Greater than 60% of the sperm must be moving actively and purposefully, and the sperm concentration should be greater than 50 million motile sperm per milliliter. The sperm morphology examination should reveal greater than 60% normal forms. Men at high risk for acquired immunodeficiency syndrome (AIDS) are excluded. Laboratory studies screen for syphilis, hepatitis B, gonorrhea, chlamydia, cytomegalovirus, and human immunodeficiency virus (HIV). It is recommended that regular donors be reexamined every 6 months. There is controversy over whether to use fresh or frozen sperm. The use of fresh sperm is associated with a higher pregnancy rate, although frozen sperm may be safer from infection. Although donors are paid, the monetary incentive is discouraged. Careful record keeping is encouraged.

There are no accurate records in the United States about how many babies are born each year from artificial insemination by donor. An estimate is 7,000–10,000 (Curie-Cohen et al. 1979). Increasingly, single women are seeking artificial insemination by donor for many reasons. These women are often in their 30s and concerned about reproductive aging, and have fears of sexually transmitted diseases and of AIDS in unscreened donor semen. Less stigma is attached to single parenthood. The feminist movement, which has stressed independence and autonomy, is now more accepting of motherhood. Single women have, however, met considerable resistance in infertility programs.

In 1980, an unmarried woman in Detroit sued Wayne State's infertility clinic when she was denied artificial insemination by donor because only married couples were accepted. She dropped the suit when the clinic began to accept single women (Corea 1979). At this time, about 10% of fertility specialists do inseminate single women (Curie-Cohen et al. 1979).

The following case illustrates the prejudice involved (Perkoff 1985). A lesbian couple who were both employed and had lived in a stable relationship for more than a decade decided they wanted a child. One woman sought artificial insemination by donor, and this procedure was done by her physician. She became pregnant and 6 weeks later was admitted to the hospital with abdominal pain. When the staff learned about the circumstances of her pregnancy, the physician, who had recently been offered a new faculty position, was denied his new job and was soundly criticized by his colleagues. There are other examples of negative attitudes (Leiblum and Barbrack 1983).

Psychological Issues

The motivations for pregnancy and for children are complex and multidetermined. The wish for a pregnancy is not always the same as that for a child. Although single women seeking donor insemination seem to be a very special group, they have some of the same conscious and unconscious reasons for wanting a pregnancy and a child as do married women. These include wanting a child to combat the fear of loneliness, to confirm one's sexual identity and bodily integrity, and to fulfill the expectations of one's parents, society, and culture. Some women long for a child to rework the relationship with their own mothers. Some may be reacting to the loss of a relationship, or a parent. Some simply want to go through this major life experience (Nadelson 1978).

Bernard (1974) wrote about single women who wanted to adopt children—"a new group" of women in their late 30s, reared in large families, often professional with good incomes who chose motherhood instead of wifehood. They chose a child instead of a husband, although they did not abandon the idea of marriage. They had succeeded in their work role and now wanted to try the mother role. Some single women choosing motherhood differed from traditional mothers in experiencing less guilt; having less self-sacrificing qualities; being less possessive; feeling that children did not owe them anything for their love; and being more androgenous in their values, more flexible, and nonfuture-oriented. They viewed marriage as more complex than motherhood.

The concern most frequently voiced about artificial insemination by donor of single women is that this represents a threat to the family and that children raised in fatherless homes will have psychological problems. There is also the fear that women may have unrealistic expectations about the qualities of sperm donors.

In the United States, however, the definition of *family* is changing (Pogrebin 1983). One in 4 children live with one parent, usually the mother, compared to 1 in 10 in 1960. Researchers estimate that 60% of today's children will spend some of their lives in one-parent homes (Kutner 1988); they are a reality of current life.

There are no long-term follow-up studies of children born to single mothers who conceived by artificial insemination by donor. There are, however, studies of children raised in homes by single mothers, lesbian and heterosexual. The major concerns are that core gender identity, sexual orientation, and future sex-role behaviors may be affected. In fact, despite theoretical formulations of psychoanalytic and social learning theories predicting that children raised in single-parent homes would have more trouble with psychosexual development, there is no support for this. Empirical studies showed that most children raised in single-parent homes with a heterosexual or lesbian parent have normal psychosexual development and may fare quite well (Cashion 1982; Golombok et al. 1983; Green 1978; Hoeffer 1981; Kirkpatrick et al. 1981; Klein 1973; Kremer et al. 1984; Strong and Schinfeld 1984). McGuire and Alexander (1985) found similar cognitive abilities in children raised in single-parent homes compared with children from two-parent homes. Gender identity and orientation are found to be normal in children raised by single mothers, heterosexual or lesbian, when there have been good parenting and social supports. Girls raised in female-headed families often have high self-esteem and achievement. Adverse psychological effects result more often from psychological disorders and lack of financial and social supports.

There are several concerns voiced by single mothers. What should the child be told about the father? How can the child be protected from peers asking about the father? How can the single mother deal with emotional stresses in raising her child alone? Are there behavioral problems in children that result from being raised by only one parent?

Children need not be told more than they can understand at any age. They should not be lied to, and should be told how much their mother wanted them. There is no way to protect them from peers other than by helping them to develop a strong sense of self-esteem. Single mothers deal with emotional stresses in raising children alone by having strong support systems.

McCartney (1985) presented psychological descriptions of 12 unmarried women requesting artificial insemination by donor at the University of North Carolina Infertility Clinic. Their motivations for seeking donor insemination were many. Some women had had infertility problems. They felt a pressure to have children while they were still capable of reproduction. They realized that they were not getting pregnant in the conventional manner and were undergoing tests and remedial procedures. When a relationship with a man broke up, they were hesitant to ask for the cooperation of a male friend who would not be the involved parent. Some women did not want the man to feel obligated to the children and some wished to have custody alone. Most women stated that they would have felt "cheap and ugly" to have had intercourse with a man they barely knew for the purpose of getting pregnant. They found adoption to be difficult for them for a variety of reasons. Adoption agencies are not usually favorably inclined toward single parents. Older children or children with problems might be available. But these women wanted infants, usually their own biological ones. These women were concerned that, even if they could adopt infants, the biological mothers may not have taken good care of themselves during pregnancy. They felt they could control their health habits during pregnancy. Finally, they firmly believed that the donors were carefully screened for genetic and infectious disorders and were therefore also healthier.

These women discussed their decisions with their parents and often co-workers, who were supportive. Ten heterosexual women enjoyed relationships with men and hoped to marry in the future. Many of the lesbian women did have a committed relationship. Most of these women had good social supports and financial security, including health insurance.

The patients seen by this author were quite similar, and stated similar concerns. The following is an example from this group.

Case History

Ms. A is a 38-year-old corporate executive very concerned about her age in relation to her childbearing status. She felt it was immoral to have sex with a man just to become pregnant without a more long and enduring relationship. A young co-worker was pregnant, and she felt envy for her. She had had a long-standing relationship with a man that had ended a year before. She considered herself heterosexual. She had continued to climb the corporate ladder and was financially very secure. She had discussed her plans for donor insemination with her mother, who was supportive. She chose a donor with physical features very unlike her living father and brother. She wished for a daughter, but a healthy child was her prime concern. This was the material from the first interview in which she sought approval for her request for donor insemination.

She was inseminated with donor sperm, became pregnant, and wanted supportive therapy during the pregnancy. She talked of her loneliness and the wish for a family. She had grown up in a family with a mother and father, but during adolescence, learned of a "secret." The man she knew as her father was not her biological father. Her mother had had a brief liaison, had gotten pregnant, and her "true father" was unknown.

As one came to know this woman better, it seemed that some of her hope was that she would have a baby to love her, to make her feel less lonely. She was depressed (dysthymic), although this was not apparent in the first interview. (She did identify with her own mother, and she accepted the fact of not having a known father.) She was able during this pregnancy to use the supportive therapy to gain more insight into her motivations, to feel less depressed, to take more control of her life, and to use her family supports in a more useful way. She hoped to marry and eventually raise her child in a two-parent home.

This case illustrates that one interview and even elaborate testing at entry into donor insemination programs may not reveal many of the issues for the women involved. This is not to suggest that there is a psychopathology that must be discovered and treated. Rather it is a suggestion that there are areas for support and also for research relevant to choices in reproduction and in parenting. Helping individuals to understand themselves better can make parenting more effective.

In summary, the women in the donor insemination programs at large medical centers were generally well educated, financially stable, and in their late 30s; sought fertility evaluations; and wanted healthy, genetically sound children before their "biological clock" ran out. They presented their relationships with others as sound. Their sexual orientations varied as did their feminist or traditional views. They did not want brief uninvolved sexual encounters, which some of them saw as "exploiting" men. They did not want custody battles. They were generally not secretive about their plans, as are many couples who have sought artificial insemination by donor because of male infertility.

Physicians and Artificial Insemination by Donor

The gynecologists who perform donor insemination usually serve as gatekeepers trying to choose individuals who will be good parents. However, a physician is a product of his or her own culture, religion, upbringing, background, and prejudices. There are no standard guidelines or preparation of physicians for this task. If medical people are not to be in charge, who should be? These questions have led to the opening of some women-controlled sperm banks on the East Coast and West Coast offering self-insemination.

At this time, considerably more research needs to be done about the attitudes and concerns and practices of physicians who perform these procedures. There is considerable stress in some of the decisions they must make. For example, should a woman bringing her own donor who is willing to be a donor but not be a parent be acceptable? Which women, if any, should be excluded?

Artificial Insemination by Donor and Legal Issues

About half of the states in this country have adopted laws relative to donor insemination or, more precisely, to the offspring of donor insemination (Andrews 1984). In Ohio in the 1950s, a bill was proposed in the legislature to punish those involved with donor insemination with a fine of $500 and 1–5 years in prison. It never passed. Most current laws since the 1960s stipulate that if the husband consents to the procedure, the child is the legal offspring of the couple. Fourteen states insist a physician be in charge of the procedure. Eleven states require filing records with the state, although confidentiality is preserved. Only Oregon has laws also stating donor insemination can be done on any woman with her written consent. No laws forbid it. Doctors often ask if they can be liable to a paternity suit by the single woman who becomes pregnant with donor insemination. The answer is no. However, in one state, a woman who had this procedure and then had a child later went on welfare. The physician who performed the procedure was chastised.

Single women have parenthood rights under the law. Single parents can adopt. Lesbians have been given custody of children, although custody has often been denied to them. Birth certificates have been a problem, but most children born to single women via donor semen insemination have a mother's name and the father is listed as "unknown."

In Ohio, as of this writing, a bill is being proposed in the legislature to allow donors to be used only one time for an insemination, to prevent future possible consanguineous marriages. It also proposes that donor information be sent to the Bureau of Vital Statistics in the child's name, with the promise of confidentiality. Many gynecologists who do artificial insemination by donor generally oppose both proposals, especially the second because of keeping records confidential.

Ethics and Artificial Insemination by Donor of Single Women

There are four possible positions in regard to these procedures (Behrman et al. 1988). First, artificial insemination by donor or by husband is wrong because masturbation, necessary to obtain the semen sample, is wrong. Sex is for procreation only. These procedures are "unnatural." Second, artificial insemination by husband is ethical, but artificial insemination by donor is not—because marriage is desirable. Anything that causes conception in marriage is acceptable. Artificial insemination by donor will affect the family unit badly and will lead to selective breeding, commercialization, and social disaster. Third is the approach that artificial insemination by donor is a medical necessity without bad effects. Fourth is that insemination by donor outside heterosexual marriage is acceptable. It is legal and is currently one of the reproductive choices for women (Behrman et al. 1988; Brody 1987).

Role of Mental Health Professionals

There is an important role for the mental health professional in the care of women choosing donor insemination, although this vital function may be filled by other suitably trained individuals or the gynecologist. First of all, the decision-making process needs careful examination of options about reproduction and parenthood. This requires knowledge about counseling, motivations for pregnancy, childbearing and child raising, and the technical aspects of the procedures. Sometimes there is an advantage in talking about the decision with a physician other than the one doing the insemination. Often, patients consider only the most positive aspects when requesting a particular technique. The counselor needs to discuss issues of confidentiality—will the woman want her thoughts shared with the gynecologist or not? The counselor should not be the gatekeeper, and sometimes this role becomes cloudy and should be clarified. The format for counseling requires some questions that each woman might ask herself. Do I want a child? How might my life be changed by having a child and raising the child as a single parent? What role did my parents play in my life and will I be the same or different? What close relationships do I have for emotional support? What financial supports do I have? Why am I choosing this method of conception? What might I tell my child about his or her father and the method of conception?

Second, the counselor can assess the individual for psychological disorders. These disorders should be treated so that decision making can be done in the most effective way.

Third, mental health professionals can consult with their gynecologic colleagues, who often face some very difficult and stressful situations in their practices.

Fourth, mental health professionals need to be involved in the shaping of legislation that is fair, equitable, and reasonable in providing access to these procedures and/or in banning procedures that are seen as exploitative.

Fifth, psychiatrists, psychologists, sociologists, nurses, ethicists, and anthropologists should be involved with their gynecologic colleagues in the study of outcomes not only of semen donor insemination, but also the many other new reproductive technologies. What are the effects on children and how are parents who underwent these procedures affected? Do counseling and support make any difference?

Artificial insemination by donor of single women is part of the reproductive technologies of our time. A considerable amount of research about psychosocial, legal, and ethical issues still needs to be done.

References

Andrews L: New Conceptions. New York, St. Martin's Press, 1984

Beck WW Jr: Two hundred years of artificial insemination (editorial). Fertil Steril 41:193–195, 1984

Behrman SJ, Kistner R, Patton G: Progress in Infertility. Boston, MA, Little, Brown, 1988

Bernard J: The Future of Motherhood. New York, Penguin, 1974

Brody E: Reproduction without sex. Law, Medicine, and Healthcare 15: 152–155, 1987

Cashion BG: Female-headed families: effects on children and clinical implications. Journal of Marital and Family Therapy 8:77–85, 1982

Corea G: The Mother Machine: Reproductive Technologies From Artificial Insemination to Artificial Wombs. New York, Harper & Row, 1979

Curie-Cohen M, Lutrell L, Shapiro S: Current practices of artificial insemination by donor in the United States. N Engl J Med 300:585–590, 1979

Golombok S, Spencer A, Rutter M: Children in lesbian and single-parent households: psychosexual and psychiatric appraisal. J Child Psychol Psychiatry 24:551–572, 1983

Green R: Sexual identity of 37 children raised by homosexual or transsexual parents. Am J Psychiatry 135:692–697, 1978

Hoeffer B: Children's acquisition of sex-role behavior in lesbian-mother families. Am J Orthopsychiatry 51:536–544, 1981

Kirkpatrick M, Smith C, Roy R: Lesbian mothers and their children: a comparative survey. Am J Orthopsychiatry 51:545–551, 1981

Klein C: The Single Parent Experience. New York, Walker, 1973

Kremer J, Frijling BW, Nass J: Psychosocial aspects of parenthood by artificial insemination by donor (letter). Lancet 1:628, 1984

Kutner L: Parent and child. The New York Times, April 7, 1988

Leiblum S, Barbrack C: Artificial insemination by donor: a survey of attitudes and knowledge in medical students and infertile couples. J Biosoc Sci 15:165–172, 1983

McCartney C: Decision by single women to conceive by artificial donor insemination. Journal of Psychosomatic Obstetrics and Gynecology 4:321, 1985

McGuire M, Alexander NJ: Artificial insemination of single women. Fertil Steril 43:182–184, 1985

Nadelson C: Normal and special aspects of pregnancy: a psychological approach, in The Woman Patient: Medical and Psychological Interfaces, Vol 1. Edited by Notman MT, Nadelson CC. New York, Plenum, 1978, pp 73–86

Perkoff G: Artificial insemination in a lesbian: a case analysis. Ann Intern Med 145:527–531, 1985

Peterson EP: New guideline for the use of semen donor insemination. Birmingham, AL, American Fertility Society, 1986

Pogrebin LC: Family Politics. New York, McGraw-Hill, 1983

Strong C, Schinfeld J: The single woman and artificial insemination by donor. J Reprod Med 29:293–299, 1984

Chapter 10

Effects of the New Reproductive Technologies on Individuals and Relationships

Leah J. Dickstein, M.D.

The Association of Women Psychiatrists, an independent organization of more than 700 members in the United States, Canada, and Europe, adopted the following resolution in Chicago on May 12, 1987: "The Association of Women Psychiatrists has expressed concerns about the potential psychological, physical, moral and genetic hazards of the new reproductive technology."

The classic text, *In Vitro Fertilization and Embryo Transfer*, contains a chapter by Wood on selection and management of patients (Wood 1984). One section includes the phrase "patient anxiety" just once in the description of general patient management in relation to time spent waiting for a laparoscopy. The words "and associated social problems" are used in regard to the mention of surrogacy; however, *no* mention is made of psychological effects or issues related to in vitro fertilization (IVF) or embryo transfer.

Although artificial insemination by donor (AID)* was first reported in the scientific literature in the United States in 1909 by Pancoast (Hard 1909),

---

Sections of this chapter were presented at the University of Louisville, Louisville, Kentucky, on March 11, 1988, during a panel on reproductive technology during Women's History Week.
*In this chapter the term *artificial insemination by donor* will include artificial insemination by the husband (homologous) and biseminal artificial insemination sperm donation by husband and male donor.

who had performed this procedure 25 years earlier in 1884 at Philadelphia's Jefferson Medical College, studies relating to these procedures have proliferated only since the 1950s. It is probably not well known that approximately 500,000 people in the United States today were born and are alive as a result of AID. This secrecy exists despite a decade of increasing media attempts to raise public awareness.

In the last several decades, as the involved reproductive techniques have become more feasible, available, and widely used, professionals in the fields of reproductive endocrinology and mental health have been faced with expected and surprising psychological repercussions in their patients and in their patients' significant others, mainly men and children. To date, least is known about the effects on children, and issues relating to men have generally been ignored or passed over quite superficially. Furthermore, although repercussions for individuals may receive some attention, even less knowledge has accumulated and been available and offered to partners concerning effects on their significant and intimate relationships.

Psychological Effects of the New Reproductive Technologies for Women

Emotional Reactions to Being Infertile

Since literature usually reflects a society's hidden as well as visible concerns, more than a dozen recent volumes on "women and literature" were reviewed, to reveal no references to the new reproductive technologies as a literary subject. Despite this topical vacuum, many psychiatrists and other mental health professionals and health professionals in general are well aware that infertility can have profound emotional effects on a woman's estimate of her gender role, sexual identity, function, and self-esteem.

After her confirmed gynecologic diagnosis, the emotionally healthy infertile woman is likely to react to her unexpected loss of fertility and her lack of reproductive choice with an initial stage of shock and a consequent barrage of varying emotions. Raised to believe that a woman's power over her body had increased with the advent of reliable birth control methods, the newly diagnosed infertile woman justifiably feels suddenly powerless. This powerlessness invades most areas of her self-esteem and affects all her usual coping mechanisms.

Her condition of infertility precipitates a number of important repercussions. The woman is likely to experience a personal identity crisis and to wonder if she is still a sexually attractive, desirable, complete, sensual woman. The implications of being and feeling defective usually include predictable reactions. Feeling defective, the woman then may feel rejection of herself by herself and commonly expects others, especially her significant other, to harbor similar feelings toward her. If she allows herself to express her self-doubts directly to her partner, he may use the opportunity to empathize and verbalize his own disappointments about *their* infertility problem, or he may reflect all the responsibility and burden onto her. If, however, she is unable or fearful to discuss with him her vulnerable—and what she labels unacceptable, shameful, and guilty feelings—then his negative emotions are likely to increase and precipitate her confusion, sexual dysfunction, a stress episode, or even an acute emotional disorder. Common resultant and reactive conditions include all degrees of depression and anxiety, including an obsessive-compulsive or panic disorder, a somatization disorder, or even psychotic or conversion symptoms—in fact, any of a myriad of psychiatric syndromes (Rosenthal 1985). Another distinct possibility is an acute or gradual withdrawal from the relationship. This relationship might previously have been described as stable, accepting, and mutually satisfying or as fragile and silently unfulfilling. The crisis of infertility can serve as the catalyst to tip the relationship's balance. After a preliminary workup reveals the likelihood of infertility, the woman, in an attempt to discover its etiology, may consent to the increasingly complicated technical procedures in the current infertility diagnostic protocol. This stepwise process usually precipitates a continuum of expectancy and hope, followed repetitively by extreme distress and negative affective reactions as each procedure takes place and reveals no correctable problem.

As with any disappointment and loss, recognition of the fact of the loss and permitting one's reaction to it are vital in the acceptance that the chances of future fertility are negligible. The woman must mourn the loss of the child or children she had fantasized conceiving with her husband, giving birth to, rearing, and having carry on their names, appearances, and traditions as well as caring for them and serving as pleasure sources in their old age (Clamar 1980).

Infertility specialists and all professionals should not expect women to proceed through this mourning period and state without professional empathy, guidance, and perhaps psychotherapy. Furthermore, women should be informed that this mourning is likely to last several years; their painful feelings may recur, particularly when they are confronted with the fact, at family gatherings and on other occasions, of having no biological children when their siblings and friends do. It should be stressed that, like all mourning experiences, one does not "get over" this loss; rather, one learns to accept and live with it.

After the mourning issue is raised, another psychological issue that must be resolved is that of the woman generally thinking and feeling that she is defective. If the organic defect resides within the woman's reproductive system, she needs education and support to accept her personal reality.

Psychological Reactions to the Process of AID/IVF

Once she has acknowledged and begun to deal with the reality of her reproductive problems, the woman then may experience other additional stresses if and when she decides to pursue the new reproductive options. Initially, second thoughts about the decision to turn to AID/IVF are common. Then she immediately wonders: will conception occur, how shall we as a couple respond, will our relationship suffer, what will others (i.e., our parents, siblings, friends, co-workers) think? Unquestionably, the woman's reactions to AID/IVF ultimately depend on the state of her premorbid mental health. The stresses of AID/IVF procedures themselves can precipitate different degrees of distress (Frank and Vogel 1988). Many women accept noninvasive investigations but fear and resist invasive laparoscopy. Other women resent the early morning rituals, often needing to be repeated for several cycles: blood tests, ultrasound, and intramuscular shots of fertility drugs. They feel ambivalent about watching their husbands still asleep or leaving for work as they leave for these unguaranteed attempts at conception. In the initial attempts at AID/IVF and embryo transfer with her husband's sperm, she often transports the sperm from home to the gynecologist's office in her brassiere to keep the sperm near body temperature. However the sperm is obtained, its insertion by the gynecologist into her reproductive system, even with her husband present, is not the setting she had envisioned for conception of their child.

Already in a heightened state of sensitivity and probably distress, she is particularly vulnerable to rejection. Her gynecologist's humaneness, professional empathy or what she perceives as psychological distance, spoken and unspoken signals, messages and mannerisms, and actual time spent with her in ongoing explanations affect her mood. The physician's office and hospital staff also become important and affect the woman's mental state. She may perceive a hurried attitude or lack of a cordial greeting and questions regarding her well-being as personal rejection, a sign of negative IVF outcome, or personal criticism. Under the circumstances of infertility, and involved in the new reproductive technologies, patients feel extremely vulnerable.

If women in therapy complain about unempathic situations, their psychiatrists and other mental health professionals should listen and encourage the women to return to their gynecologists and to speak directly to them about their perceived reactions and to voice what they do want (i.e., an appropriately empathic response). If the patient is reticent to do so, her psychiatrist can offer to intervene. It is well known that we all feel differently, not only when in possession of useful knowledge, but also when our interactions with powerful others occur in the context of mutual respect and professional empathy.

The woman may also experience strong ambivalence, not only about accepting her husband's or unknown donor sperm in an artificial circumstance, but also understandable ambivalence about all the procedures. Thoughts range from the idea that perhaps with a different husband or at an earlier age she would not have been forced to seek this option, to consequent guilt feelings and anger about her self-described outlandish and irrational thoughts. Extreme although common fantasies surface about "having a secret affair" to become pregnant if the woman believes or is told the problem rests with her partner.

Another basic psychological issue that must be recognized is that of feelings about confidentiality about the procedures and about taking time off from work for the involved appointments. Secrecy surrounding the entire process adds another unexpected burdensome dimension. Realistic maintenance of privacy in some instances and unnecessary secrecy in other situations should be discussed, whether raised by the patient, couple, or professional.

While the woman may decide not to tell family and friends, she must give some valid explanation for her ongoing absences, for up to several hours, to her employer and to her co-workers. Furthermore, she may have to inquire into the company's employee health insurance policy to see if any of these IVF procedures are covered. In addition to the issue of health insurance coverage for the procedures, the issues of salary, personal leave time, lunch hours, or even accrued vacation time to cover these absences must be discussed since this is not a one-time event. The woman may decide to tell her immediate supervisor and workers responsible to her and ask them in turn to keep the matter confidential. These decisions may appear perfunctory and/or trivial to professionals; nevertheless, confidentiality or revelation are not unimportant issues. If the woman herself does not raise them, the psychiatrist should and must add that these are expected additional stresses to the technical situation itself.

Although co-workers usually share in the details and stages of celebration of a worker's, or spouse of a worker's, pregnancy and birth of a child, the same situation usually does not apply to IVF. Because of the likelihood of ongoing absences, co-workers, staff, or supervisor may also harbor resentment and frustration for being overburdened while they simultaneously offer support and empathy to the woman and her efforts. It is incumbent on the psychiatrist to encourage the woman to verbalize these potential feelings at work to minimize unconscious retribution.

Confidentiality also concerns the name on the child's birth certificate. Beneath all of these concerns, there is the anxiety-provoking issue of if, how, what, and when to tell the wished-for child of the circumstances of its conception. The psychosocial pros and cons about the birth certificate parental names have lifetime repercussions. Although our current culture is increasingly accepting of the new reproductive technologies, one cannot predict responses two decades hence. However, there must be concern for the future young adult's reaction to his or her out-of-the-ordinary birth certificate information and also conception. Young children ask each other, and teachers and other school, camp, health, and recreational staff ask children aloud, about names and information on certificates. IVF parents may also be confronted by adolescents, intensely concerned about body developmental transitions and body image, wondering why they do not look like anyone "on either side" or upset when told "your father's sperm or your mother's eggs were not able to be used."

Since access to medical and other types of records is constantly increasing, it appears sensible to advise IVF patients to plan on revealing appropriate information with clear explanations to their children at appropriate times in the children's lives. The contraindications to revealing information include identifying these children as differing in conception from "everyone else." If sperm or eggs were donated for the IVF procedure, this additional information would have to be shared, and the child-adult over a lifetime would need to come to terms with this, and, if appropriate, seek help in doing so.

Admitting to herself that she may want this baby to fulfill her perceived gender role in society can be another stressor for the infertile woman. Is she attempting to gain finally her parents' elusive acceptance and love, or that of her in-laws, religious group, her husband, or herself? How strong is her need to please others propelling her into this technological, expensive, and perhaps tenuous procedure? Does she feel an overwhelming need to imitate peers? Is competition with siblings, friends, and co-workers an issue? Does she feel she owes her parents grandchildren? Is she simply attempting to meet a girlhood goal she always expected to achieve? Questions such as who wants this child and for what apparent reasons are a sensitive aspect of the infertility workup usually ignored by professionals and patients alike.

Everyone interested in conception ruminates about birth defects; these are additional legitimate stresses for AID/IVF women who wonder if the unnatural process and unknown donor may increase risks of birth defects. Often suppressed is the uncertainty regarding the ability to love the child as she might have if conception had been "natural." As AID/IVF become more openly acknowledged, fewer anxieties may arise for all involved parties, both before and after a successful pregnancy. However, professionals must note that psychological difficulties may not cease with the child's birth. The woman must be warned that future concerns may arise about the child's identity, mental and physical health, and development and interpersonal attachments, especially in the nuclear family. These concerns under certain circumstances can escalate to crisis level. Alternative solutions should be envisioned by the couple and discussed over time as the child ages. All these possibilities should be raised in the preparatory sessions to IVF. Patients should be counseled by their gynecologists and, if in therapy, by their psychiatrists that many of these issues are an inevitable part of the process. Patients must accept these issues and be responsive to their potential surfacing as they accept the IVF technology. Once more the couple should be supported to understand that professional help can always be sought.

The importance of the woman's premorbid mental health has already been mentioned. It is interesting to note that psychological testing is considered part of the surrogacy procedure, yet it is not commonplace with AID/IVF. Psychiatrists, obstetricians, and couples involved in surrogacy who require psychological testing of the surrogate mother are clearly and justifiably concerned about her mental health, yet they appear to ignore this issue of mental health in the case of the IVF woman and sperm donor man. Whether this discrepancy is another unrecognized gender issue and whether psychological testing to identify mental fitness should be mandated in every instance are important questions for future research. There have also been no studies to date that deal with the possibility that these new reproductive technologies might exacerbate an individual's emotional problems if she were either to complete or be denied this procedure. The enormous professional responsibility to evaluate and rule on such selection is in some sense similar to research already accumulated about organ transplantation.

In one study of 340 AID women, 6 were diagnosed as psychologically ill (Guttmacher 1960). From an impressionistic viewpoint, AID outcomes generally indicated remarkably good psychological health in mothers. For the AID woman, bearing a biological child meets several narcissistic needs concerning fulfillment of her sex and gender roles. If the woman is immature or emotionally unstable, she can act inappropriately with a superior attitude toward her infertile significant other. Even with discussion early in the AID process about sex role, the consequence and reality can still precipitate episodes of confusion, self-doubt, sexual dysfunction, and all the disorders mentioned earlier.

Psychological Effects of the AID/IVF Experience for Men

This section on psychological effects for men is also thoroughly discussed by Myers (Chapter 3, this volume). However, in the past three decades, psychiatric researchers and clinicians have found it very useful and enlightening for newer gender issues to be discussed by both male and female professionals to raise and discuss issues from all possible vantage points. The two authors, therefore, encourage the male and female reader to consider this issue of the gender of the researcher when reviewing material presented.

Involvement in a new reproductive technology can be very stressful for the fertile man and even more so if he is the infertile partner. Sex-role socialized to be virile and proud of it, men in the early years of research in the new reproductive methods never underwent physical evaluation until "their women" had preceded them and had been found to be reproductively competent. Professional and patient usually expected it was the woman's problem and were surprised when the organic abnormality was found in the male partner. Only then were the men invited, encouraged, and supported during their investigative procedures. The men's psychological discomfort usually exceeded their physical discomfort. In some instances, men refused evaluation, especially when it involved an invasive procedure such as repair of a varicocele, and the women accepted this response without retort or confrontation. However, since research has proved that 40% of infertility problems emanate from males, and that evaluation of men's reproductive functioning is easier and simpler than women's, most men's reluctance has decreased and their initial involvement has increased (Shapiro 1988). This constructive change in attitude and practice has in essence rotated the infertility problem from a woman's problem to a more realistic couple's problem.

The process of masturbation to obtain sperm samples for diagnosis and for conception can be difficult for the man. Personal preconceived as well as cultural views of masturbation may affect his ability, willingness, and comfort with this procedure. Whether he performs at home or in one of the physician's offices can add to his stress, and this must be acknowledged and discussed. At times he "forgets the dates" when he is supposed to produce a sample because he is "busy at work" or he does not specifically and verbally acknowledge his wife's repeated daily early-morning office visits for blood tests, ultrasound procedures, and shots. Then he must deal with the direct and indirect, legitimate and exaggerated repercussions of her angry and sad feelings toward him.

Another important psychological concern of men is that of donor sperm in biseminal artificial insemination. Apart from the woman's and the couple's fears and discomfort, the man's legitimate emotional pain, shame, anger, curiosity, and gratitude toward this virile "lucky" other man must be acknowledged and resolved, first for himself and definitely for the couple and future child. Since men's difficulties expressing vulnerable emotions are now generally well known to stem primarily from sex-role socialization and possibly from biological predisposition, infertility specialists must raise these normal feelings during the very first investigative interview. Empathic, direct confrontation and acknowledgment by the professional of normal poignant emotions will facilitate a man's continuing involvement in the workup and fertilization process. Ignoring these vulnerable feelings can send messages that they are unusual, unacceptable, and of little value and that discussing them is needless and only appropriate for those who need psychiatric care.

If the infertility problem resides in the woman, a man must face his conflicts over thoughts of "what if I had a different wife" and "lost" children. As with women in similar circumstances, men's feelings and fantasies must be acknowledged necessarily to themselves and before involvement in IVF. When appropriate, both partners as a couple can work through their infertility problem, disappointments, and acceptance of this alternative procedure. The man must also recognize the importance of his ability to communicate his circumstance of involvement with a new reproductive technology with his nuclear family, co-workers, superiors, and friends. Even though women and men have been marrying at later ages in the past three decades than had been the custom and a significant percentage feel freer to choose to abstain from childbearing, cultural expectations still abound that all adults who are able will become parents and that men will care for, support, and protect their wives and children. For men as well as for women, fertility as an issue may also be raised when adults in their 30s and 40s seek promotion, transfer, and new career opportunities, and their personal lives become potential areas of interest for prospective employers.

Psychological Effects of the New Reproductive Technologies for Couples

Effects of the new reproductive technologies for couples are numerous and both negative and positive. A basic issue that must be raised in the initial physician contact is that the couple is infertile regardless of which adult has an identified abnormality. This fact will need ongoing clarification and restatement as the individuals come to terms with their long-held hopes and beliefs and their current reality.

It is important that all professionals accept and assist patients in the realization that each partner in the couple proceeds at a different pace of desiring and accepting some form of AID/IVF. Usually these important individual differences and consequent lag times in acceptance or reluctance to proceed are unknown and/or unrecognized by both partners because they simply do not communicate with each other. Overshadowed and overwhelmed by personal feelings about themselves and the entire unexpected extraordinary fertilization process, each has assumed the other knows and understands the partner, when obviously this is not the case. Once personal concerns are verbalized and differences are acknowledged, a sense of relief becomes obvious in both partners, and direct communication, clarification, and negotiation can begin.

Then, as the decision for and the process of AID/IVF begin, both individually and together, the couple must become aware of and work through "what went wrong" in the process of attempting natural conception. Was there hysterectomy, oophorectomy, or orchitis because of infection, cystic disease, endometriosis, or other abnormal growth processes in adolescence or in young adulthood? Was there lack of or inadequate sperm? Is the reason for infertility still unidentifiable? Was it because of earlier sexual or other behavior and seen as "retribution" in the eyes of some? Where applicable, the couple must resolve feelings about donor insemination. Who is this anonymous donor? Why did/would he donate sperm? Why would she donate an egg? What is his or her personal, family, medical, and psychiatric history? Often a first and legitimate concern is what he or she looks like. Will my child look only or more like him or her? How will our appearances blend? Will our genetic factors mix well or cause a genetic problem? Will we ever meet the donor? Will we recognize the donor because of our child's features? Will we simply pass by sometime? Will we stop him? Will he look at our young adolescent and wonder about lineage? Will our adolescent notice the stranger because the latter has features shockingly similar to the adolescent at an age when concern about whom we resemble is normal? Will our young adult ever ask questions? What will he or she want to know? When will this occur? How should we respond?

Those questions are natural, obvious, and better recognized early and verbalized and discussed than denied. Forethought must be given to whether many of the questions should ever be broached with the developing adolescent and young adult as they face medical, including psychiatric, issues and problems in future years.

One researcher raised the specter of participants' fear of future incest because of donor anonymity (Rubin 1965). As part of the complete explanation of the IVF procedure, the gynecologist should mention the normal concern about possible incest and, at the same time, reassure the couple that gynecologists in most states maintain confidential records of the sperm and egg donors, and if the question arose at a later date when the IVF child proposed marrying, records could be checked (Notman 1984).

Both partners may need to seek intensive, insight-oriented individual therapy for newly recognized or chronic psychiatric symptoms. Each partner must rework personal circumstances, life events, and rationalizations that allow her and him eventually to resolve their frustration, anger, sadness, guilt, and doubts. Only then can they reach concordance and go forth with the 20th century's miraculous technologies that offer them the opportunity to have a child biologically related to at least one of them. As psychiatrists, we would hope that, ideally, most adults resolve within themselves and in their relationships the discordance between their long-held goals, aspirations, and dreams and the current realities of their lives. In therapy, IVF patients need encouragement, support, and time to resolve the multitude of disappointments related to their infertility.

A second important issue to identify initially and early in the physician-patient relationship is the separation for the couple of sexuality and sexual desires and satisfactions from their procreative capacities. A third issue for the couple is how they handle the longed-for pregnancy and others' comments, jokes, and unknowing remarks. In usual circumstances, others' remarks are well meant and well received. In the circumstance of AID/IVF, the couple will do better to discuss between themselves beforehand how they may feel and respond to other's remarks. If the couple appear to be distressed or coping poorly, expedient physician referral to a mental health professional is necessary.

Two studies of 58 (Levie 1967) and 127 (Jackson 1957) AID couples followed over 11 years report extremely encouraging results. The children tested above average mentally and physically, and the couples' marriages were rated as consolidated and improved. Other clinicians have recommended that couples seeking AID not proceed with psychological testing (Waltzer 1982). One 7-year follow-up study of 800 AID marriages led to only one known divorce (Behrman 1975). These researchers theorized that "the AID secret," the couple's prior deliberations about the procedure, and their personal mental health keep them successfully together.

There are several encouraging reports regarding positive AID results. In one study (Berger 1982), successful AID/IVF recipients stated they chose AID because they 1) wanted to experience a pregnancy; 2) were dissatisfied with adoption procedures, including the length of waiting and approval time and the questions they were asked; 3) saw benefits from maternal or paternal heredity; 4) felt a closer relationship with the child than if they had chosen the adoption procedure; and 5) saw AID as a way to conceal their infertility problem. Several researchers reported studies that revealed that more than 96% of AID couples said they would select AID/IVF again (e.g., Levie 1967).

Psychological Effects of the New Reproductive Technologies for Children

Little rigorous research is available concerning AID children born since 1976, when the use of these technologies became more commonplace. The children may never question their biological parents' identities unless they are informed directly or learn accidentally about the unusual circumstances of their conception. However, if they do learn about their different biological origins, rearing parents and even the involved physicians should be ready and available to respond to questions and understandable feelings. Concerns about biological parents' medical histories are always appropriate and important. If there are siblings, their parental connections will need explanation.

Several psychiatrists have recommended that for the children's sake, no one be told about the use of AID/IVF (e.g., Waltzer 1982). Waltzer defended his view by stating that this secrecy is in the child's best interests and that if and when the child learns about the conception, difficulties will ensue. On the other hand, I agree with Shapiro (1988), who recommended that the young adolescent be told in an appropriate manner at an appropriate time because family secrets can be "corrosive." This knowledge, like knowledge of family history of adoption, suicide, alcoholism, and schizophrenia (to name a few of the important hidden stigmata in many families), is another unusual and vital part of this young person's unusual life. If parent-child relationships are healthy, this information will be accepted and handled well.

An Australian follow-up study of 50 couples who received donor sperm because of male infertility found no major emotional problems when the AID children were between 1 and 3 years old (Mushin et al. 1986). When interviewed, 34 of 50 couples planned not to tell the child and verbalized a high request for a repeat AID experience. A follow-up study of 216 AID mothers and children revealed fewer problems than with adoptions (Haman 1959).

From a Clinical Vantage Point

The following observations are representative of more than a decade of professional involvement with women and men seeking AID/IVF.

A psychiatrist, on behalf of a professional woman whose AID child was 2 years old, asked me to intercede and speak with the sperm donor to gain knowledge about the donor's personal and family medical history as well as information about his appearance, interests, and personality. The obstetrician had the donor, a resident in one of our university training programs, contact me. He knew me, although I did not recognize his voice, and with knowledge of the request, he readily complied by giving the information. He asked no questions about the child, who, I had already been told, was developing normally and happily and resembled the maternal grandfather.

Another couple proceeded through all of the available tests with no identified problem. The woman sought personal therapy, the man turned to alcohol, and, after several years, they divorced. Their unresolved personal problems, together with their unexpected infertility, stressed the relationship beyond their willingness or capacity to cope without couple therapy, which was refused.

A different couple, with prior personal issues resolved in individual therapy, willingly sought couple therapy when they realized that infertility was a reality and their independent coping strategies not sufficient. In psychotherapy, they faced their childless future and verbalized all the disappointments ahead: no parent-child activities, no tumultuous adolescents who would remind them of themselves, and no worries about young adults and cars, dating, weddings, and grandchildren. After they appeared to accept these disappointments, they began to identify what they could look forward to and might enjoy individually and together. They mentioned hobbies, volunteering, projects to help others, their work, and their concern for and satisfactions with each other. Again and again they were encouraged to voice their pain, life's unfairness, and their personal strengths and coping mechanisms. Beyond redefining their personal and mutual new life goals, they addressed how they would relate to family, friends, and acquaintances.

During the period of couple therapy, they were also strongly encouraged to attend Resolve meetings (discussed later) to learn first hand how others coped. Although they did not become pregnant, their relationship remains happy.

Finally, another example reflects contact with two professionals who sought psychiatric assistance and assumed the patient role. In this instance, simultaneous ongoing therapy for both individuals and for the couple was advised to deal with considerable personal unresolved developmental issues that were affecting the couple in their current attempts at coping and complying with the infertility workup and strategies. Intermittent contact with treating psychiatric and other medical professionals was also found useful to the infertility specialists and beneficial to the couple. From the beginning therapy sessions, it appeared to the psychiatrist that one partner needed to deal with unresolved guilt and mourning over one parent's death and the other parent's chronic illness, loneliness, and dependency. This same partner was encouraged to face personal unresolved dependency issues and reasons for low self-esteem. A number of sterotypic gender roles and issues became apparent and were worked through. The second partner also recognized residual anger and the need to please both a demanding and narcissistic parent and a depressed, distant parent. This partner also had gender issues to resolve relating to communication problems and emotional openness. As the two individuals progressed independently, they became more at ease in facing *their* infertility problem and willingly accepted the psychiatrist's offers to contact a local IVF specialist, as well as one who was nationally recognized. Their therapy extended over a 3-year period. They had not realized initially the need for the process but voiced gratitude at termination. At that time, they appeared ready and able to continue IVF attempts and to keep in touch with the therapist.

Another obvious factor is economics. To date, a large number of the adults interested in AID/IVF are college educated and can economically afford the technology. Since most of the procedures are not covered by insurance, the considerable costs must be borne individually. Savings must be accumulated in advance, and the participants should discuss for what these funds might have originally been earmarked. Ongoing discussions and negotiations must occur as the number of attempts increase and potential economic hardships and sacrifices are made or plans are altered.

The Mental Health Professional's Role

The enormous amount of professional understanding, empathy, tact, patience, support, and education required by adults involved in the new reproductive technologies must be recognized, first as legitimate and second as necessary and time consuming (Seibel 1988). Nonphysician mental health professionals should work together with psychiatrists and other medical specialists on patients' behalf in the initial AID/IVF process. Psychiatrists are in the unique position of being able to understand and explain medical procedures involved in the gynecologic steps that comprise IVF. It appears appropriate then that psychiatrists should assume responsibility for initial evaluations and explanations for IVF patients, and that other mental health professionals as well as psychiatrists be responsible for psychotherapy. IVF teams might consider including a psychiatrist as consultant and director of a mental health group of psychologist and social worker therapists.

Psychiatrists particularly interested in psychological issues related to IVF can contribute in major ways to the maintenance of good mental health in all involved in these procedures. On-site training programs to relieve anxiety and counseling and support programs led by social workers are worthwhile (Edwards and Purdy 1982). Patients, as well as gynecologists, their staffs, and other health professionals, would benefit from meeting with a psychiatrist to be made aware of the psychological reactions and problems a majority of patients and their partners, as well as staff and professionals, may experience through their involvement with IVF (Greil et al. 1988). Educational small and large meetings centered in hospitals, academic department clinics, private group practices, and community groups would offer psychiatrists the opportunities to share issues and respond to questions and concerns. This educational service would support everyone's interests and needs and would enable professionals at all levels to be more understanding and supportive to patients and their significant others.

Since most women who seek IVF do not also seek psychiatric or other mental health care, psychiatrists might want to develop brochures or booklets that discuss issues addressed in this chapter, which could be distributed in gynecologists' offices. Awareness that one's feelings and fears are common and expected can reduce distress and anxiety.

The psychiatrist involved in close professional practice with infertility specialists, or whose patients seek this treatment, might offer to meet jointly with the gynecologist and the couple. When couples embark on their plan to conceive, they do not expect additional psychiatric problems. If one or both are already in treatment, their therapist may foresee acute exacerbations or further progress because a decision has been made and a process has begun. Professionals have noted different outcomes following AID: several published opinions clearly indicated that adoption was preferable, and concluded that a decision to participate in AID is itself indicative of emotional disturbance (e.g., Sokoloff 1987). Since studies in the field are just emerging in near-critical numbers and results often conflict, psychiatrists working with patients selecting AID/IVF should individualize therapy and recommendations. Difficulties arise regarding AID/IVF because previously unidentified and unresolved problems require psychotherapeutic work.

The success of local chapters of the consumer advocacy group Resolve (Menning 1984) is well known. Resolve, a national organization for infertile adults founded in 1973 in Massachusetts by Barbara Menning, offers infertile couples access to information, peer support, and professional speakers (Menning 1977). Psychiatrists interested in infertility might wish to consider attending a local Resolve meeting as a speaker or as a guest to gain more insight.

Discussion

An important issue beginning to surface involves donor selection in AID. Although obstetricians attempt to match recipients' and donors' appearance, one might question, if records are maintained, whether couples should be allowed to select donors as they do surrogate mothers. Consequent psychological effects might then include donors' or their spouses' reluctance to donate sperm or eggs, and if donation occurs, then the complications from the donors' interest in "their" eventual child and their spouse's jealousy, anger, emotional pain, and curiosity about unknown children. Beyond the financial factor for the donors, other issues such as proving one's fertility, helping humanity, and building self-esteem may be involved.

Clearly *all* health professionals must recognize the importance of and potential for negative psychological consequences of AID/IVF in their patients. Professionals should share with patients the fact that the occurrence of psychological problems for parents and children is unpredictable and that long-term psychological and emotional consequences have yet to be identified and addressed.

At present, simultaneous research and clinical protocols must be developed to identify and describe stressors and problems unique to IVF patients. Adding to the outcome studies already available, especially from Australia, valid information concerning the most effective treatment methods at various stages of infertility investigation and IVF procedures is vital.

Although incest among IVF children seems improbable, careful data collection and retention should be maintained over the next four decades to validate this hypothesis and concern. Benefits and risks of psychological testing of IVF participants must be evaluated.

Studies of IVF children and their relationships and self-esteem are further subjects requiring investigation. Questions not yet commonly raised in the literature but certain to occur, simply from increased knowledge of genetics and the importance of role modeling in the environment, are: Will the IVF children themselves, as adults, require and be likely to request IVF technology for themselves? Will they require and request it more or less frequently than non-IVF-conceived adults?

As with every new technological procedure, research questions that could not even have been postulated will arise in the next decade. Thoughtful interventions by psychiatrists, other mental health professionals, infertility specialists and their staffs, and the patients themselves can mitigate numerous problems. Like all new technologies, the abuse of IVF must be foreseen and guarded against. IVF abuse may include multiple pregnancies of multiple births in families unwilling or unable to parent the offspring appropriately; the use of women's eggs and their men's sperm implanted in poor women living in third world countries to "save the bother of pregnancy"; IVF technology to breed offspring having otherwise impossible combinations of superior physical and intellectual prowess; and even more remote, still unvoiced immoral objectives. As the Association of Women Psychiatrists stated in their 1987 resolution, what has offered life, love, and joy to some should not be at the expense of others.

References

Behrman SJ: Artificial insemination, in Progress in Infertility. Edited by Behrman SJ, Kistner RW. Boston, MA, Little, Brown, 1975, pp 779–789

Berger DM: Psychological aspects of donor insemination. Int J Psychiatry Med 12:49–57, 1982

Clamar A: Psychological implications of donor insemination. Am J Psychoanal 40:173–177, 1980

Edwards RG, Purdy JM (eds): Human Conception In Vitro: Proceedings of the First Bourn Hall Meeting. London, Academic, 1982

Frank D, Vogel M: The Baby Makers. New York, Carroll & Graf, 1988

Greil AL, Leitko TA, Porter KL: Infertility: his and hers. Gender and Society 2:172–199, 1988

Guttmacher AF: Role of artificial insemination in the treatment of sterility. Obstet Gynecol Surv 15:781, 1960

Haman JO: Therapeutic donor insemination: a review of 440 cases. California Medicine 90:130, 1959

Hard AD: Artificial impregnation. Med World 27:163, 1909

Jackson MH: Artificial insemination (donor). Eugenic Review 48:205, 1957

Levie LH: An inquiry into the psychological effects on parents of artificial insemination with donor sperm. Eugenic Review 59:97–105, 1967

Menning BE: Infertility: A Guide for the Childless Couple. Englewood Cliffs, NJ, Prentice-Hall, 1977

Menning BE: Resolve, in Infertility: Medical, Emotional, and Social Considerations. Edited by Mazor MD, Simons HF. New York, Human Sciences Press, 1984

Mushin DN, Berreda-Hanson MC, Spensley JC: In vitro fertilization children: early psychosocial development. J In Vitro Fert Embryo Transfer 3:247–252, 1986

Notman MT: Psychological aspects of AID, in Infertility: Medical, Emotional, and Social Considerations. Edited by Mazor MD, Simon HF. New York, Human Sciences Press, 1984

Rosenthal MB: Grappling with the emotional aspects of infertility. Contemporary Ob/Gyn, July 1985, pp 97–105

Rubin B: Psychological aspects of human artificial insemination. Arch Gen Psychiatry 13:121, 1965

Seibel MM: A new era in reproductive technology: in vitro fertilization, gamete intra-fallopian transfer and donated gametes and embryos. N Engl J Med 318:828–834, 1988

Shapiro SA: Psychological consequences of infertility in critical psychophysical passages in the life of a woman, in A Psychodynamic Perspective. Edited by Offerman-Zuckerberg J. New York, Plenum Medical, 1988, pp 269–289

Sokoloff BZ: Alternative methods of reproduction: effects on the child. Clin Pediatr (Phila) 26:11–16, 1987

Waltzer H: Psychological and legal aspects of artificial insemination (AID): an overview. Am J Psychother 36:91–102, 1982

Wood C: Selection and management of patients, in In Vitro Fertilization and Embryo Transfer. Edited by Wood C, Trounson A. Edinburgh, Churchill Livingstone, 1984, pp 175–188

Chapter 11

Gender Differences in Counseling Needs During Infertility Treatment

Cheryl F. McCartney, M.D.
Cicilia Y. Wada, Ph.D.

Being infertile and undergoing modern treatment for the condition create stress for the individuals in an infertile couple and for their relationship. The infertile partner feels abnormal, betrayed by his or her body, and responsible for the loss of potential childbearing for the couple. The partners often keep their infertility a secret and thus depend solely on each other for support (Lalos et al. 1985; Menning 1980). Although treatment options for infertility have increased in number and complexity, they have several common psychological impacts. They expose couples' most intimate experience—their sexual lives. They can be costly in terms of money, time investment, and, for some, experiencing painful procedures. Several treatments require couples to examine their moral values to decide if a treatment that is technologically possible is "right" (e.g., artificial insemination by donor, surrogate parenting, ovum donation). Since most techniques have a significant

This research was supported in part by USPHS General Research Support Award 5-S01-FR-05406 and by the Kenneth D. Dickinson Memorial Fund.

We acknowledge the helpful contributions of Luther M. Talbert, M.D., Robert F. Conry, Ph.D., Pamela M. Smith, R.N., Jo Anne L. Earp, Sc.D., Cynthia Hedricks, Ph.D., Annette Rykwalder, M.P.H., William H. McCartney, M.D., and Sandra Stinnett, M.S.

failure rate, couples must decide together when to stop treatment if no pregnancy occurs. Adjustment to childlessness is another emotional challenge for couples who have not conceived.

Psychological disturbance secondary to infertility is more frequent among women than men. Freeman et al.'s (1985) work with in vitro fertilization candidates showed that while 49% of the women considered infertility the most upsetting experience in their lives, only 15% of the men felt this strongly.

A woman's adjustment to infertility is improved when she has a confiding relationship with her spouse (McEwan et al. 1987). In fact, several authors asserted that the emotional distress of infertility is a couple's problem and should be addressed in marital counseling (Hendricks 1985; McCartney 1985; Menning 1980). Since it has been reported that 22% of infertile couples already had marital problems prior to treatment (Seastrunk et al. 1984), and that treatment is known to produce additional stresses, it is clear that effective detection of relationship distress and referral of affected couples for counseling is an important role for infertility clinics.

Although patient surveys indicate interest in psychological counseling for the stresses of infertility and its treatment (Daniluk et al. 1985; Owens and Read 1984), referral rates for these interventions are low. Daniluk et al. found that 53% of men and 72% of women beginning infertility treatment would have participated in counseling if it had been available. Many couples applying for in vitro fertilization after several years of standard infertility treatment retrospectively expressed their wishes for early discussion of their concerns and feelings (Freeman et al. 1985; Lalos et al. 1985). But in a clinic where all new infertility patients were offered counseling, only 29% accepted the referral (Bresnick and Taymor 1979). At the University of North Carolina Infertility Clinic, where patients are not routinely referred, only 2% of the couples requested counseling services.

One possible explanation for this low referral rate, suggested by Mahlstedt (1985), is that patients often hide emotional pain from physicians because they are self-conscious about their feelings and sensitive about the medical staff's anticipated criticism of them for being troublesome. Some patients may fear that further infertility treatment will be withheld if they admit any emotional distress.

Another hypothesis to explain these findings is that there is a difference between men and women partners' perceptions of the distress in their relationships, which interferes with their ability to seek help as a couple. The study discussed in this chapter compares male and female attitudes about actions to relieve relationship distress of infertile couples. By studying patients' satisfaction with the doctor-patient relationship, it attempts to define a role for the physician in detecting relationship distress and referring couples for counseling.

Materials and Methods

Measure

A 67-item questionnaire was designed based on interviews with infertility clinic staff and patients, as well as formal psychiatric consultations and psychotherapy with infertile women and couples. Content validity was determined by review with former patients, psychiatric colleagues, and clinic staff. Fifty statements focused on six topics: patient education, sharing the infertility secret, clinic attention to men's emotional needs, attention to the couple's relationship, treatment stresses, and the doctor-patient relationship. Four possible responses were arrayed as a Likert-type scale and ranged from 1 (strongly disagree) to 4 (strongly agree). Three open-ended items requesting written comments were answered by about one-third of respondents. Fourteen items elicited demographic data and pregnancy and treatment history.

The initial 559 questionnaire packets were mailed to all women who had attended at least two infertility clinic appointments in the previous 18 months. They had undergone pharmacologic ovulation induction, artificial donor insemination, or microsurgical reanastomosis of fallopian tubes (the most advanced techniques available at the time). They had either achieved pregnancy (39%), terminated treatment with no pregnancy (31%), or were still actively in treatment with no pregnancy (30%). Each packet contained two identical instruments: one for the woman and one for her partner with the request that they respond independently. A second wave of questionnaires were sent to nonresponders. Of the 1,118 questionnaires sent, 486 (43.5%) were returned (56% of those who had become pregnant, 27% of those who had stopped treatment, and 57% of those who were still actively in treatment). The responders consisted of 269 (48%) women and 217 (39%) men. The response rate for the subgroup with male infertility was 49% (92 individuals). This report deals with the 203 couples (406 subjects) for which responses were received from both partners.

Subjects

Demographic characteristics. The respondents were female patients and their male partners in a university-based infertility practice. Like the target population, they were older and better educated than usual expectant parents. The median age of women was 30.5 years and that of men was 31.8 years. Two-thirds of the men and women had college or postgraduate training. A majority had professional occupations and combined annual incomes greater than $25,000.

Classification variables.   Classification variables concern the couple's pregnancy and treatment history. The first classification variable is prior fertility. In one group of couples, one or both members had been biological parents in the past. Prior to entering the infertility clinic, only the woman in 23 (11.3%) of the couples, only the man in 13 (6.4%), and both partners in 27 (13.3%) had already been biological parents. (This distribution in the study population is comparable to that of the overall infertility clinic population.) Of these prior pregnancies, 13% had resulted from previous infertility treatment.

The second classification variable is the gender of the infertile partner. The woman was the infertile partner in 161 (79.3%) of the couples. The man was infertile in 42 (20.7%) of the couples.

The patients' high motivation to become pregnant was demonstrated by the time they had invested: 55.7% had been trying to conceive for more than 2 years *before* entering the clinic.

The third classification variable is the duration of treatment in the clinic. Duration of treatment was less than 1 year for 120 couples (59.1%), 1–2 years for 62 couples (30.5%), and more than 2 years for 31 couples (15.3%).

The fourth classification variable is the outcome of treatment. Of the couples, 61 (30.1%) achieved pregnancy, 16 (7.9%) achieved pregnancy but lost it before delivery of an infant, 79 (39.1%) were actively in treatment when they responded to the questionnaire, and 46 (22.7%) left the clinic without achieving pregnancy.

Data Analysis

Because the questionnaire included many items, missing data were expected. An initial exploration was done to ascertain whether there were patterns of nonresponse that might create a bias in the results. At least one data value was missing for 33% of respondents, but it was determined that the distribution of missing data was not related to any particular group of respondents. Thus the mean value of the responses to a given question, calculated separately for each gender, was imputed to those respondents with missing values.

To consolidate the data, image factor analysis, with Harris-Kaiser oblique transformation (Harris and Kaiser 1964), was employed and performed separately for each gender. Factor analysis is a standard statistical technique that groups the questionnaire items into fundamental dimensions. Four factors that explained most of the variation in the data, both for men and women, were determined. The factor *distress* involved questions about patients' feelings of relationship distress, including feelings of tension in the relationship before and during treatment, sexual dysfunction, feelings of isolation, and consideration of divorce. The factor *willingness* was composed of items indicating patients' willingness to take independent action to improve their emotional comfort during treatment, such as interest in reading about infertility, talking informally by telephone to other patients, and joining a professionally led support group. The factor *openness* included items asking about patients' openness to relationship counseling, such as interest in being interviewed in the clinic about their relationship, having counselors available at the clinic, and interest in seeking relationship counseling if distress developed. The factor *satisfaction* contained items requesting patients' opinions about whether the doctor got to know them as a person and whether doctors explained the meaning of tests, anticipated treatments, and costs. Prestudy pilot interviews had indicated that these issues contribute to patients' satisfaction with the doctor-patient relationship.

Factor scores were the unit of analysis. These were computed as the average of the responses to the items that comprised each factor and were computed for each gender based on the factor analyses done for men and women.

The objectives of the statistical analysis were to examine 1) the relationships among factors for each gender and between genders, 2) gender differences with respect to factor scores, and 3) the effects of the classification variables on factor scores for each gender.

The relationships among the four factors were examined using Pearson coefficients of correlation. An overall correlation between each factor score, separate correlations among all factors within genders, and correlations between genders for each factor were performed.

Paired *t* tests were used to determine the significance of gender differences for each factor.

One-way analysis of variance was used to assess the effects of the classification variables on factor scores. When a significant effect was found, pairwise comparisons (*t* tests) between all levels of the classification variable were examined to determine which levels differed with respect to the factor score mean. This analysis was done for each gender and then for a score computed as the gender difference in factor scores for each couple.

Results

Correlations Between Factors

The correlation coefficients between factors for women and men are shown in Table 1. In both genders, there were significant correlations ($P < .01$) between distress and willingness, distress and openness, and willingness and openness. For men only, openness was significantly negatively correlated ($P < .05$) with satisfaction. Correlations between male and female factor scores were significant ($P < .01$) for distress (.493), openness (.285), and satisfaction (.502), but not for willingness (.069).

Table 1.   Correlations between factors by gender

Factors	Correlation coefficient	
	Women	Men
Distress–willingness	.249*	.301*
Distress–openness	.348*	.346*
Willingness–openness	.473*	.376*
Distress–satisfaction	.026	–.125
Willingness–satisfaction	.127	.085
Openness–satisfaction	.087	–.159**

*$P < .01$. **$P < .05$.

Gender Differences in Factor Scores

Table 2 displays mean factor scores for each gender and the gender differences in scores. Women scored significantly higher than men ($P < .001$–.002) on all four factors.

Effect of Classification Variables on Factor Scores

Table 3 shows the results of the analyses of the effects of each classification variable on factor scores for each gender and for the differences between genders. Duration of treatment and outcome of treatment were the only significant classification variables, and they affected openness and satisfaction. Figure 1 illustrates that while with all treatment outcomes women were more open to counseling than men ($P = .01$), the greatest differences between the genders occurred in the groups who achieved pregnancy (.34) and those who ended infertility treatment without pregnancy (.32). These differences were statistically significantly greater than the gender differences of the

Table 2.   Means (±SE) of factor scores by gender

Factor	Gender	Mean ± SE	P
Distress	Female	2.16 ± 0.029	
	Male	2.05 ± 0.028	
	Difference	0.11 ± 0.029	<.001
Willingness	Female	2.89 ± 0.017	
	Male	2.81 ± 0.019	
	Difference	0.08 ± 0.025	.002
Openness	Female	2.80 ± 0.026	
	Male	2.56 ± 0.024	
	Difference	0.24 ± 0.031	<.001
Satisfaction	Female	2.85 ± 0.021	
	Male	2.60 ± 0.022	
	Difference	0.25 ± 0.021	<.001

Table 3. Effect of classification variables on factors by gender

Factor	Classification variable	P Women	Men	Difference
Distress	Prior fertility	.574	.561	.936
	Gender infertile	.318	.508	.696
	Duration	.538	.630	.815
	Outcome	.486	.920	.761
Willingness	Prior fertility	.729	.171	.764
	Gender infertile	.251	.102	.626
	Duration	.267	.117	.702
	Outcome	.386	.731	.828
Openness	Prior fertility	.096	.654	.390
	Gender infertile	.268	.971	.322
	Duration	.632	.499	.863
	Outcome	.197	.197	.010*
Satisfaction	Prior fertility	.840	.582	.153
	Gender infertile	.283	.668	.137
	Duration	.005**	.003**	.890
	Outcome	.011*	.013*	.400

*.01 < P < .05. **P < .01.

groups who were in active treatment (.14) and those who had gotten pregnant but lost the pregnancy (.10). Men and women expressed significant decreases in satisfaction with the doctor-patient relationship with increasing duration of treatment (Figure 2). For durations of <1 year, 1–2 years, and >2 years, satisfaction means were 2.89, 2.85, and 2.66, respectively, for women and 2.65, 2.59, and 2.40, respectively, for men. For both genders, pairwise comparisons indicated a significant reduction in satisfaction between <1 year and >2 years and between 1–2 years and >2 years. Satisfaction was significantly affected by outcome for both men and women (Figure 3). For the outcomes of pregnancy, pregnancy lost, active treatment, and terminated treatment with no pregnancy, the satisfaction means for women were 2.93, 2.84, and 2.84, and 2.74, respectively, and for men the means were 2.71, 2.59, 2.55, and 2.54, respectively. For women, the factor mean for satisfaction was significantly less for the group who terminated treatment than for the group who got pregnant. For men, the means during active treatment and at termination were both significantly less when the outcome was pregnancy.

Discussion

The results of this questionnaire survey of infertile couples show that while some emotional reactions to infertility treatment are shared by women and men, there are some gender differences in degree and timing of their reactions. These differences are important because they may interfere with the

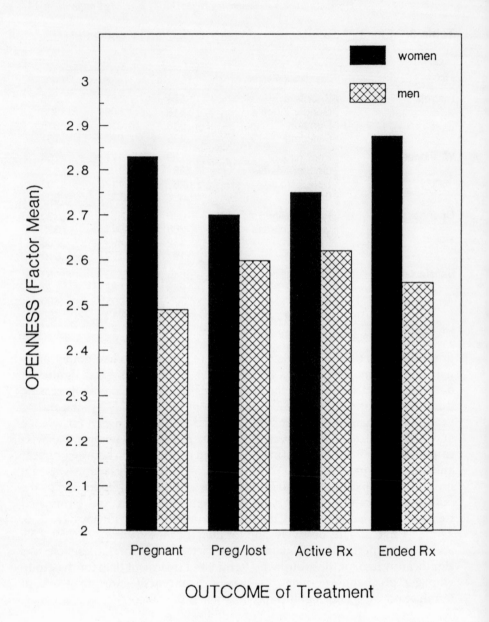

Figure 1. Openness by outcome for each gender.

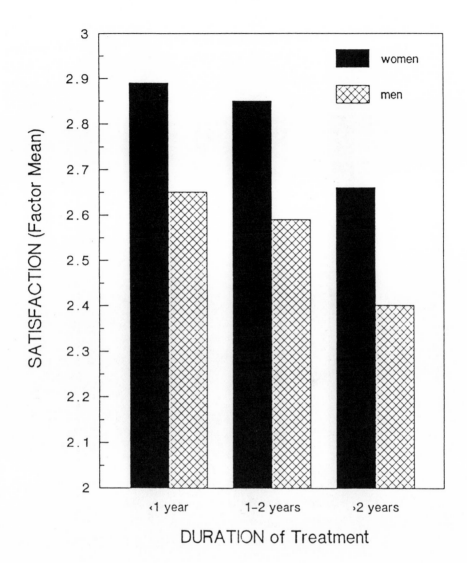

Figure 2. Satisfaction by duration of treatment.

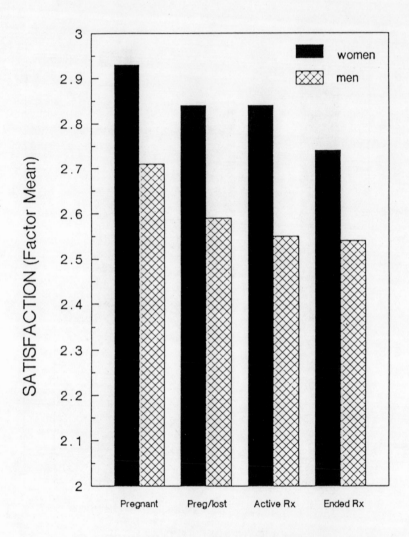

Figure 3. Satisfaction by outcome for each gender.

partners' ability to agree about taking actions to protect and/or repair the emotional health of their relationships.

As expected logically, the study shows that, for both genders, increasing relationship distress is correlated with increasing willingness to take independent action toward relief of that distress, and with increasing openness to a specific action: seeking professional counseling as a couple. Satisfaction with the doctor-patient relationship is not related to distress or willingness; however, for men only, openness increases as satisfaction decreases (and vice versa).

Between genders, distress, openness, and satisfaction are correlated, but willingness is not. This suggests that members of couples experience variations in these factors in a similar direction, even though they may differ in intensity of feelings. However, partners may be quite different in their enthusiasm for actions—such as reading, talking to other infertile people, or joining support groups—which could reduce the experience of stress caused by infertility.

Each factor focuses on relationships, either with the partner or with the doctor. For each, women score significantly higher than men. There are several explanations for this. First, the woman's body is the object of the treatment, even when the man is the infertile partner. Her active participation in procedures and her frequent direct contact with the physician and clinic staff lead to a more intense reaction for her than for her partner.

A second explanation can be found in the theory of the gender differences in sex-role socialization. Women are raised to value the development and nurturance of relationships, whereas men are taught to prize the achievement of goals (Klein 1983). Thus it is possible that women see infertility as a threat to relationships with husbands, parents, and unborn children, whereas men see it as a failure to achieve a life goal. The partners' differing perceptions of their distress, with the accompanying differences in feelings of urgency to relieve it with relationship counseling, can lead to marital discord. Clinical experience indicates that a woman may feel misunderstood and thus isolated just at the time when effective communication is vital. For example, a man may either press his partner to pursue treatment beyond her tolerance (to achieve his goal of pregnancy) or urge her to discontinue treatment before she can accept infertility, if he is not able to empathize with her distress. She may perceive his pressure as devaluation of her worth as a partner and believe that a pregnancy is, for him, a condition for continuing the marriage. In addition, solving emotional problems by psychotherapy, which uses a relationship model, is likely to be more attractive to women than to men.

Although women indicate more openness overall, the outcome of treatment seems to be an important influence on the size of the difference between men's and women's openness to relationship counseling. The greatest gender disparity occurs at end points of treatment intervention: pregnancy or termination of treatment without pregnancy. Thus it would be useful for doctors to probe for evidence of relationship distress in the couple at these points and to suggest counseling if indicated, since the couple will be unlikely to reach consensus independently about seeking help from a mental health professional.

Both genders indicate decreasing satisfaction with increasing duration of treatment. Both indicate less satisfaction when therapy ends without pregnancy than when pregnancy occurs. In a descriptive paper, Hertz (1982) theorized that infertile women changed their perceptions of physicians when pregnancy was not achieved from "surrogates for an ideal, strong, protective father" to "aggressive and active male figure(s) posing an existential threat to the patient as he attempts to 'bring about changes' in her" (p. 97). He explained that the peak of deterioration of the physician-patient relationship occurs when the woman begins to project her guilt and internalized anger onto the physician. Although part of the explanation for decreased satisfaction may be due to the patient's internal psychological reactions, there is likely also to be a contribution by the physician to the changed relationship. Patients may correctly perceive their doctors' disappointment, feelings of personal inadequacy, and less optimistic attitude, which may lead to decreased intensity of engagement in the doctor-patient relationship. The study findings suggest that to avoid ending treatment with the double disappointment of unchanged infertility and an unresolved doctor-patient relationship, physicians must acknowledge with patients the possibility of treatment failure and must initiate discussion about a realistic end point for treatment.

Regarding men's role in offering emotional support to infertile wives, representative responses from the open-ended items in the questionnaire indicate that men are aware of their partner's distress and are receptive to learning how to be more helpful to them. To the questionnaire statement, "At times my partner needed more comfort than I could provide," 57% of the men responded with agreement. To an open-ended question, one man wrote:

> I think the male should be enlightened as to the effect infertility has on women. Even though it may be a joint problem, the woman seems to bear the brunt of the load of disappointment and depression. I personally underestimated the impact it was having on my wife. . . . Men should be encouraged and taught how to share the problem of infertility.

Another commented:

> Most of the experience of infertility was experienced by me in the role of support to my wife. That was a very difficult role to play without knowledge of the reality of problems, treatments' possibilities for success, etc. The clinic could help lessen

the extent of anguish in an infertile wife by developing some helps for a supportive, but ineffectively directed husband.

The findings must be interpreted with some caution because of the problems associated with mailed questionnaire surveys. There is a differing response rate between men and women and among patients with the different treatment outcomes. Subjects in groups not in treatment at the time of the study recorded memories of feelings, rather than current feelings. This analysis selected the subgroup of patients in which both partners in a couple responded. These could be considered the most psychologically interested subgroup, and thus it is possible that gender differences could be even greater than reported here in subjects whose male partners declined to respond.

In summary, this questionnaire survey of infertile couples confirms that women perceive more relationship distress than men and are more open to counseling. It suggests that physicians should inquire about relationship distress at intervals during treatment because couples are unlikely to reach consensus about the need for counseling without this intervention. To protect the support offered by a satisfactory doctor-patient relationship, physicians should collaborate with couples to acknowledge that treatment may not produce pregnancy, to determine the optimal amount of treatment to attempt, and to plan a termination point if pregnancy is not achieved.

References

Bresnick E, Taymor ML: The role of counseling in infertility. Fertil Steril 32:154–156, 1979

Daniluk J, Leader A, Taylor PJ: Psychological Aspects of Infertility. Paper presented at the annual meeting of the American Psychiatric Association, Dallas, TX, May 18–24, 1985

Freeman EW, Boxer AS, Rickels K, et al: Psychological evaluation and support in a program of in vitro fertilization and embryo transfer. Fertil Steril 43:48–53, 1985

Harris CW, Kaiser HF: Oblique factor analytic solutions by orthogonal transformations. Psychometrika 29:347, 1964

Hendricks MC: Feminist therapy with women and couples who are infertile, in Handbook of Feminist Therapy: Women's Issues in Psychotherapy. Edited by Rosewater LB, Walker LE. New York, Springer, 1985, pp 147–158

Hertz DG: Infertility and the physician-patient relationship: a biopsychosocial challenge. Gen Hosp Psychiatry 4:95–101, 1982

Klein R: Gender identity and sex-role stereotyping: clinical issues in human sexuality, in Treatment Interventions in Human Sexuality. Edited by Nadelson CC, Marcotte DB. New York, Plenum, 1983, p 63

Lalos A, Lalos O, Jacobsson L, et al: A psychosocial characterization of infertile couples before surgical treatment of the female. Journal of Psychosomatic Obstetrics and Gynaecology 4:83–93, 1985

Mahlstedt PP: The psychological component of infertility. Fertil Steril 43:335–346, 1985

McCartney CF: The doctor-patient relationship in infertility treatment, in Infertility: A

Practical Guide for the Physician, 2nd Edition. Edited by Hammond MG, Talbert LM. Oradell, NJ, Medical Economics Books, 1985, pp 15–24

McEwan KL, Costello CG, Taylor PG: Adjustment to infertility. J Abnorm Psychol 96:108–116, 1987

Menning BE: The emotional needs of infertile couples. Fertil Steril 34:313–319, 1980

Owens DJ, Read MW: Patients' experience with an assessment of subfertility testing and treatment. Journal of Reproductive and Infant Psychology 2:7–17, 1984

Seastrunk JW, Kemery TD, Adelsberg B, et al: Psychological evaluation of couples in an inpatient reproductive biology unit. Fertil Steril 41:97S, 1984

Chapter 12

Psychiatric Research and the New Reproductive Technologies

Jennifer Downey, M.D.
Mary McKinney, M.A.

What can research tell us about the potential psychological impact of the new reproductive technologies? Clinical experience and intuition tell us that innovative procedures, such as artificial insemination, gamete intrafallopian transfer, in vitro fertilization, and the use of surrogate gestational mothers must place new stresses on all the individuals involved. But are there discrete symptoms, patterns of distress, or psychiatric disorders that might be expected to develop in certain cases? Researchers have yet to assess the implications of the latest advances in reproductive medicine. Many of the techniques are new, the number of couples receiving such treatment is relatively small, and, most critically, the variables that would likely affect psychological reactions are so numerous, complex, and intertwined that any one study can give us only a tiny section of the emotional picture. Indications for seeking such new treatments, previous tests and treatment received, financial costs, physical health, social status and other demographic variables, the marital relationship, ethical and legal ramifications of medical innovations, social pressures to bear children, prior adjustment to the issue of potential infertility, and personal coping styles—all are factors that may positively or negatively affect an individual's response to the new medical interventions available. The impact of these factors on individuals and couples needs to be studied.

What we know at this point about psychological responses to the use of medical interventions that assist reproduction comes mainly from studies of people who have sought treatment for a fertility problem or who sought to avoid genetic transmission of a familial illness by resorting to artificial insemination or embryo transfer. To date, difficulty conceiving has been the most common indication for using the new reproductive technologies. Now, however, the pool of patients to be treated is increasing as individuals request the new procedures for social reasons. Single women may request artificial insemination with donor sperm; married women may wish to use a surrogate to avoid the experience of pregnancy; and couples may use amniocentesis to determine the sex of the baby, with abortion requested if the fetus is not the preferred gender. With the exception of artificial insemination of the single woman (Rosenthal, Chapter 9, this volume), little is known about the individuals who seek help from physicians for social reasons. This will be an especially difficult area to investigate since, in many cases, admitting nonmedical reasons for treatment would cause the service to be withheld.

A patient's reasons for seeking reproduction-enhancing treatment are crucial because attitudes and feelings about preexisting medical conditions will be inextricably entangled with the patient's response to whichever procedure is used. It is important to remember that most reasons for seeking these treatments are perceived as deficits: the couple's inability to conceive, the lack of a partner, or abnormal genetic makeup. Thus the findings we will discuss result from the combination of perceiving oneself as having a deficit and experiencing the treatment. Both illness and potential cure have psychological impact.

What Has Been Done

The Scope of Infertility as a Problem

Infertility, by the accepted medical definition of a year or more of unprotected coitus without pregnancy, is a common health problem. Medical authorities such as Speroff et al. (1983) estimated that 10–15% of couples will be affected. The only population-based study of infertility in women, the National Survey of Family Growth, found that of all currently married couples in the United States in 1982 with a wife 15–44 years of age, the percentage of infertile couples was 13.9% among those who were not surgically sterile (Hirsch and Mosher 1987). In addition, as Hirsch and Mosher noted, there is increasing demand for infertility treatment because of postponement of childbearing, increases in the proportion of infertile couples seeking care, a shrinking supply of adoptable infants, new techniques for treating infertile couples, and increased public awareness of these treatments.

Intact reproductive capacity is usually taken for granted until tested by opportunities to achieve pregnancy that do not lead to conception (Miller 1981). The point at which it registers on an individual that he or she may have a fertility problem, and therefore may be unable to have biological children, is a point of intense stress and threat to self-esteem (Menning 1980). The problems infertile people may have with the identity of disability, a "spoiled identity" as Matthews and Matthews (1986) called it, are compounded by the sense of social stigma they experience. Miall (1986) found that more than one-half the women she studied who were involuntarily childless hesitated to tell others about it, two-thirds answered questions in a deliberately vague way, and nearly one-third lied about it. There is suggestive evidence that identity as an infertile person is unconsciously rejected also. For instance, Cella and Najavits (1986) found that of men treated for Hodgkin's disease with radiation and chemotherapy (which leaves 80–90% infertile), and who said they wanted to have children in the future, 38% failed to bank sperm before undergoing treatment, although all had been advised to do so. Of the men who failed to bank sperm, 93% said they had believed that they would remain fertile.

Stresses of Infertility: Uncertainty and Loss

An infertile couple experience many losses: of potential children; of genetic continuity; of a life goal; of the experiences of pregnancy, childbearing and breast-feeding; and of control over their own bodies (Valentine 1986). Yet the experience of infertility is frequently not recognized as one of loss, since the mourning is for a potential rather than an actual child. Failure or inability to grieve over infertility is among the most common problems seen clinically, in part because uncertainty is a factor in most diagnoses, unless the man is azoospermic (without sperm) or until the woman reaches menopause. Thus Yogi Berra's comment about a baseball game —"it's not over 'til it's over"— applies particularly to the infertility experience. A couple may undergo multiple tests and treatments for years, then suddenly conceive. For a sizable number of patients, only passage of time will demonstrate whether they are irreversibly infertile or not. This situation makes grieving for the never-existent child (and one's poorly functioning body) more difficult to resolve.

The process of undergoing fertility evaluation and treatment constitutes an additional life stress because the procedure deals with intensely personal matters (sexual functioning) and may be protracted, intrusive, expensive, and painful. For example, a simple regimen most women are advised to follow—taking their basal body temperature every morning before getting out of bed—ensures that they will think about their fertility over and over.

Even a test as simple as the postcoital semen analysis is associated with increased rates of impotence and ejaculatory incompetence in men (Keye 1984) and anorgasmia in women (DeVries et al. 1984). Berger (1980a, 1980b) found that more than 60% of the men he studied experienced transient impotence after being diagnosed as azoospermic. While a disappointing diagnosis may cause dysfunction, the cost and effort required of patients by elaborate treatments, such as in vitro fertilization, seem to raise unrealistic hopes. For instance, although candidates for in vitro fertilization are routinely counseled that fewer than one of five couples achieve pregnancy with the procedure, the majority opting for in vitro fertilization believe that they will somehow "beat the odds" and conceive (Leiblum et al. 1987). Psychiatric symptoms after trying "heroic" interventions are frequent. Mao and Wood's (1984) follow-up study of patients who discontinued in vitro fertilization treatment without conceiving found that 60% of patients reported anxiety and 48% reported depression as important reasons for discontinuing treatment.

A fertility problem may also become a focus for marital conflict if the partners do not share the same motivation for pregnancy or use the same coping strategies. Most studies suggest that women admit to more distress than men (e.g., Keye et al. 1981; McEwan et al. 1987), but it is unclear whether this means that women are more profoundly affected or simply more willing to admit to symptoms. A significant proportion of women who have no fertility problem, but who have partners who are infertile, nevertheless lie to friends and family, saying that they themselves have the problem (Czyba and Chevret 1979). This willingness to assume public responsibility can be construed as indirect evidence that infertility and feelings about it are viewed as less socially "acceptable" in men than in women. Berger's (1980a, 1980b) data on the high incidence of impotence in men who are informed they are azoospermic surely suggest that infertility affects them profoundly, leaving the possibility open that men deny being more affected for defensive reasons. Clinicians report differences in psychological response depending on who is the partner with the anatomic abnormality, with unaffected partners expressing anger and affected partners expressing guilt and even the conviction that their spouses should leave them for someone else who is fertile (Bresnick 1984; Mazor 1984; Menning 1980).

Psychological Difficulties in Infertility Patients: Cause or Consequence

The pain, guilt, and anger over having a body deficit and deficit as a couple and the stress of tests and treatments are factors that have potential repercussions on the fertility patient's psychological health. How such issues are related, however, is unknown. So far there has been little research that helps separate causal factors from consequences. Three decades ago, psychiatric approaches to infertility focused on psychogenic factors as a cause of infertility for the 30–40% of couples in which no organic problem could be found. Today, with improved diagnostic techniques, an organic abnormality and presumed etiology can be established for more than 90% of all couples seeking fertility treatment. With this refinement in diagnostic capabilities, the number of conditions that can rightfully be attributed to "psychogenic infertility" has shrunk. Currently recognized psychological problems that cause infertility include infrequent or exclusively nonvaginal intercourse, amenorrhea secondary to anorexia nervosa, and conditions requiring the use of medications (e.g., major tranquilizers) that may inhibit ovulation. Other psychiatric disorders, such as anxiety or depression, could possibly affect fertility via a hypothalamic or pituitary mechanism, but this has not been established to date.

With this reassessment of the role of the mind in causing infertility has come reassessment of the role of mental health professionals in treating patients with fertility problems. There are no well-designed and executed studies that demonstrate that psychological treatment enhances conception as an outcome in the general fertility patient population. Clinicians have suggested (Bresnick and Taymor 1979; Rosenfeld and Mitchell 1979) that couples undergoing fertility evaluation and treatment may benefit from the availability of counseling services to assist in coping with the life stress involved, and significant numbers of patients when queried indicate that this would be helpful (e.g., Daniluk 1988). However, there is currently no evidence indicating better psychological outcome in patients who receive these services (Edelmann and Connolly 1986), and many professionals note that only a small percentage of couples receiving fertility treatment avail themselves of proffered psychological help, although they endorse its availability for others.

The Time Factor: Infertility as an Ongoing Experience

Fertility problems and their psychological repercussions are frequently experienced over a period of years, yet we know of only a few studies that have evaluated subjects at more than one time. Morse and Dennerstein (1985) assessed 30 couples presenting for in vitro fertilization, but at the 2 months' posttreatment follow-up assessment, only 53% responded. One couple had conceived, and the remaining patients seemed deeply distressed by their failure. Lalos et al. (1985a, 1985b, 1986) studied 24 infertile couples before and after the woman's reconstructive tubal surgery and found that partners' feelings for each other had worsened and their sex life had deteriorated after 2 years. At follow-up, both men and women complained equally of grief, but the women were more likely to complain of emotional symptoms, such as irritability, fatigue, and depression. About 70% of the couples had neither succeeded in achieving pregnancy nor tried to obtain another solution to the infertility problem, even though they had been told that if they did not conceive within a year after surgery, chances of later pregnancy were slight. Overall, the couples seemed to be doing significantly worse 2 years later.

Snarey et al. reported (1987) a post hoc analysis of fertility data from a 40-year longitudinal study of boys of urban blue-collar origins. Of 343 married men assessed at age 47 years, 52 (15.2%) had experienced infertility in their first marriage. Of the couples, 44% chose to keep trying rather than to adopt, 31% remained childless, and 25% chose adoption. The investigators reported that infertile men initially coped with their childlessness by "substitute parenting" the children of others (25%); a nonhuman object, such as a car or a pet (63%); or themselves, by becoming preoccupied with activities such as bodybuilding or health foods (13%). The men who engaged in substitute parenting activities with others' children were most likely to adopt and most likely to achieve "generativity" in later life (a concept from Erikson [1950, 1975], who defines it as a life stage in which one establishes and guides the next generation). Adoption was *least* likely for those couples who had spent more than 8 years trying to have a child. The investigators suggested that years of anxiety and effort may have exhausted these infertile couples and left them feeling that they were behind where they should be in the socially defined life-cycle. Overall, the study showed that while the infertility problem could be handled in a number of ways, resolution of the problem made the achievement of generativity more likely.

In addition to the work of Snarey et al. (1987), we know of only a few other studies that have included both a control population and baseline measures of psychological functioning in their research design. In one such investigation, Paulson et al. (1988) found that, on referral to a fertility clinic, 150 patients showed no significant differences in personality profiles or on measures of anxiety and depression when compared to 50 volunteer controls recruited from college, graduate, and nursing programs and from gynecologic practices. Similarly, in a comparison of 153 fertility patients and 141 fertile controls, Freeman et al. (1983) also found no difference in baseline psychological self-assessment measures. Using a subset of this subject group to study drug-induced ovulation, the researchers (Garcia et al. 1985) employed a double-blind, crossover trial of clomiphene citrate and a placebo. Of 49 fertility patients, half were randomly chosen to begin treatment with clomiphene and half were given a placebo. The groups were switched after five treatment cycles. At the end of the study, 11 subjects had achieved pregnancy during clomiphene treatment and 3 during placebo treatment. The investigators also tested the possible relationship of psychological factors with the ability to conceive by giving each subject a battery of emotional, behavioral, and personality inventories before beginning the drug regimen. When baseline measures of psychological factors were later compared, no significant psychological differences were found among the women who had achieved pregnancy and those who did not conceive.

Although baseline measures of psychological functioning showed no differences between ultimately successful and unsuccessful fertility patients in the Garcia et al. (1985) study, it seems clear that eventually the emotional state of these two groups must vary greatly. Those who are unsuccessful must accept their inability to conceive, which constitutes an additional life stress since, at that point, one's own biological children must be grieved as lost for good. Accepting infertility, and considering alternative life strategies such as adoption, is a process complicated by the rapid developments in medical treatment, which change what is defined as irreversible infertility. A study by Collins et al. (1983) found that 41% of 597 couples treated in a university fertility clinic became pregnant during the 7-year course of the study. However, the percentage of couples who conceive is rising as both diagnostic and therapeutic capabilities improve.

Questions Raised by New Treatments: Ethical and Legal Issues

The hope offered by advanced fertility-enhancing technologies has put patients with severe fertility problems in a kind of limbo—How will they choose among the panoply of available treatments, some experimental, expensive, and with varying degrees of societal and legal sanction and protection? The Ethics Committee of the American Fertility Society (1986) described treatment strategies such as the use of surrogate mothers and surrogate gestational mothers (women who gestate a genetically unrelated embryo) as "clinical experiments," that is, innovative procedures whose consequences must be examined before they are made generally available. There are also potential legal and social ramifications for all those involved in artificial insemination. As Sokoloff (1987) pointed out, only 28 states have passed laws stating that the offspring of artificial insemination by donor is the legal child of the sperm recipient and her consenting husband. Given the legal and ethical ambiguities involved in procedures such as artificial insemination by donor and in vitro fertilization and the lack of information about long-term consequences, infertile couples must weigh many risks when they decide whether to elect these treatments. The wealth of opportunity constitutes a stress in itself since couples are less and less likely to be advised to stop treatment, and the quest for pregnancy may stretch into decades. There is also the threat that these procreative opportunities may be withdrawn if legislative regulation and control increase.

Even from the limited amount of data available, it is clear that there is psychological risk for some men and women undergoing reproductive interventions. Which individuals are at risk, during which phases of treatment, and given which added external stressors are more difficult questions to answer. Some interventions may turn out to be so psychologically stressful that they should not be made available without psychological and legal safeguards. Yet, given the inconclusive findings of research conducted so far, providing the new fertility-enhancing treatments responsibly so as to minimize adverse psychological sequelae is still a matter of intuition and guesswork.

What Needs to Be Done

The Importance of a Longitudinal Approach

To evaluate the psychological impact of the latest reproductive interventions, we need to assess the mental health status of patients over time. At the outset of their quest to conceive, very few people are considered for advanced technologies, and one would expect attitudes and emotions to shift at points before, during, and after successful, or unsuccessful, interventions. Diagnostic evaluation takes time, and usually there is a series of increasingly ambitious procedures as the simpler, less expensive, and less hazardous treatments are tried. Evaluating couples at a single point in time makes it impossible to assess the severity of perceived psychological difficulties relative to a baseline. Unlike miscarriage, which is a discrete, stressful event, the failure to conceive is a non-event, often experienced over years. Although it seems likely that there will be many changes in couples' attitudes toward the problem—depending, for example, on the stage of the workup—it is not even known at this time whether patients presenting for initial fertility evaluation commonly feel hope and a sense of relief from taking action, or intense anxiety and dysphoria. We believe, as Edelmann and Connolly (1986) have written, that prospective, longitudinal studies are needed to assess how patients and their spouses are affected over time and to assess which combination of factors is most likely to lead to clinically significant levels of distress.

In the course of time, many couples will drop out of fertility treatment, either because they conceive, because they adopt, or because they find the medical interventions too stressful. Other fertility patients may quit because they divorce, run out of money, grow too old, or decide they want to devote more time to their careers. To date, many of the patients studied have had years of unsuccessful treatment and represent a highly selected group. Are they the survivors—unusually healthy, persistent, and rich? Or do they lack the flexibility shown by couples who adopt or adjust to a childless marriage? Most studies conducted so far have assessed a heterogeneous group of individuals followed at a fertility clinic and therefore have been unable to compare couples who will continue indefinitely as fertility patients with those who will drop out of treatment without achieving fertility.

Who Should Be Studied: Choosing Subjects and Controls

Selection of subjects and control groups is one of the most difficult tasks faced by responsible researchers. As noted above, the definition of "fertility patient" changes over time, and subject criteria must be thoughtfully chosen. As longitudinal studies are implemented, adequate control groups become particularly important, since over time a certain percentage of the sample will develop psychiatric symptoms and disorders for reasons unrelated to fertility. In theory, finding an adequate control group is a simple matter; in terms of actual research design, however, it poses a challenging problem. What group of people would constitute an adequate control group for people receiving treatment using the new reproductive technologies? Edelmann and Connolly (1986) suggested comparing women receiving fertility treatment with women anticipating the birth of their first child, because both groups are experiencing stressful reproductive life events. In a longitudinal study of female fertility patients we are currently conducting at Columbia Presbyterian Medical Center (Downey et al. 1989), we elected to use as controls age-matched women who are using contraception and coming for routine gynecologic care to the same practitioners. Neither of these choices is ideal. Women having a first child experience radical life changes, many of which are physically apparent and publicly sanctioned, unlike the hidden stresses of infertility. Women presenting for routine care may have different values, ambitions, and partner relationships than women of comparable age seeking fertility treatment.

Choosing subjects for studies of this kind raises a number of issues. At the most basic level, the results of psychological studies of couples applying to in vitro fertilization programs demonstrate that investigators in this field cannot be affiliated with the gatekeepers for scarce treatments. In these studies, couples have reported remarkable mental health and marital adjustment, an expected phenomenon given that psychological health was used as a screening criterion. Choosing subjects also means choosing whom to eliminate: certain studies in the past have dropped fertility patients who achieve pregnancy because they no longer have a reproductive problem, an example of data lost through less than optimal research design.

A critical gap in research involving individuals with fertility concerns has been the failure to study the male partners of the women presenting for fertility treatment. We do not think this is wholly because the gynecologist is usually the one who coordinates the fertility workup, with a urologist used as needed as a consultant, although no doubt this contributes to the problem. Men are much more reluctant than women to discuss any problems related to reproductive failure, even in a clinical setting, let alone as research participants. Studies designed to assess couples have demonstrated that the woman is sometimes the only partner willing to participate (McEwan et al. 1987; Valentine 1986). Studies in the future must elicit men's participation. The use of male interviewers may help here.

Another gap in our knowledge is the lack of information about the many individuals who never present for reproductive treatment but nevertheless are involuntarily childless. Hirsch and Mosher (1987) presented data suggesting that a large proportion of women with secondary infertility who do not seek treatment are of low socioeconomic status and that middle- and upper-class women are overrepresented among users of fertility-enhancing interventions. In part, this is because fertility treatment has been most available to patients who can pay for it out-of-pocket. As medical insurance begins to cover the cost of fertility treatment, however, women in modest circumstances will request it. There are, of course, many nonfinancial reasons why childless couples may not seek treatment, and a community-based study is needed to assess mental health effects of infertility in these men and women.

In general, the subjects of infertility studies have been treated as though they were a homogeneous group, which obscures the adverse psychological impact infertility may have on certain subsets of patients. As larger studies are conducted, researchers will be able to make finer distinctions among subjects. In addition to assessing fertility patients by the length of time they have been trying to achieve pregnancy, and by which phase of testing and treatment they are undergoing, it will be important to divide the subject pool by medical diagnosis. Women receiving medications such as danazol and human menopausal gonadotropins may report different physical and psychological symptoms than women treated without drugs. Undiagnosed problems may increase feelings of helplessness: McEwan et al. (1987) found that women who had not yet received a diagnosis were much more distressed than women who had.

Besides the couple who are receiving the reproductive intervention, there are a number of other affected individuals who will require further study—for example, the donors of the gametes and the surrogate mothers, whether or not they contribute eggs. Initial studies of these subjects include the work of Parker (1983), who found that surrogate mothers are motivated by several complementary factors including financial need, the desire to be pregnant, the wish to give the gift of a baby to an infertile couple, and the desire (often unconscious) to master unresolved feelings about a previous abortion or voluntary relinquishment of a baby. Reame (1987) found that 75% of the surrogate mothers she studied experienced at least moderate symptoms of perinatal loss and grief at the time of relinquishment of the newborn.

Among the affected individuals who need to be studied are the offspring of successful fertility treatment. Clinically they appear often to be "special" children from the very beginning, just as are children who were born very premature and spent long periods of time in the hospital, and who are still being called "my preemie" by their mothers 25 years later. So far, follow-up studies of children conceived via in vitro fertilization suggest that the majority of these children are achieving normal developmental milestones, with most problems associated with twinning, cesarean delivery, and low birth weight due to preterm delivery (Mushin et al. 1986; Spensley et al.

1986). Children conceived by donor insemination are also at risk for later psychological sequelae because of family secrecy concerning their parentage and the sense of deficit experienced by their nongenetic fathers. In a study of 43 couples who successfully conceived using artificial insemination by donor, and whose children ranged in age from less than 1 year to 9 years old, 17 reported maintaining total confidentiality about the fertility treatment (Leeton and Blackwell 1982). The remaining 26 had told only one or two close friends or relatives. In this same sample, 84% of the couples did not plan to tell their children about their anonymous parentage. In a group of couples seeking donor insemination for a second child, Milsom and Bergman (1982) found that only 1 of 92 couples planned to tell the children the truth about their conception. There are potential hazards in trying to maintain total secrecy about artificial insemination by donor. Clinicians report that sometimes during the heat of a divorce or other family crisis a parent will blurt out the information to a child in a harmful way (Sokoloff 1987).

What Should Be Studied: Methodological and Theoretical Issues

In addition to the need for the implementation of longitudinal studies, a more careful selection of both subjects and controls, and a greater range of subjects, a fourth issue that future research needs to address is the severity of psychological symptoms that occur during reproductive interventions. Patients in a number of studies report symptoms (e.g., depression) in response to infertility or its medical treatment. However, feelings of depression, which may be an appropriate reaction to the stress of infertility, must be distinguished from depression as a diagnosable mental disorder. The tendency of patients to attribute any negative mental health experiences to a concurrent life problem (in this case, infertility) is a pitfall for investigators. It is natural to look for precipitants, but the fertility issue is so intertwined with self-esteem, body image, sexuality, marital satisfaction, life goals, and societal norms that correlations can rarely be distilled into simple formulas of cause and effect. As mental health professionals, we have a particular responsibility to deal carefully with the issue of distress versus dysfunction because our findings are often read by physicians who are not versed in psychiatric diagnostic criteria and to whom the distinction between a symptom and a mental disorder may not be clear.

Several other methodological components need to be incorporated into future research designs in the field. Ellsworth and Shain (1985) pointed out that researchers need to consider several methodological issues: the use of placebo groups whenever ethical, crossover designs to determine which factors are both significantly and independently associated with outcome variables, and increased sample sizes with emphasis on attrition and participation rates. Another important strategy is the use of standardized self-report questionnaires in conjunction with interviews by trained clinicians, rather than relying on a single assessment procedure as has often been done in the past.

Finally, researchers of the future in this field must grapple with the choice of an adequate theoretical perspective. Failure to conceive or inability to bear a living child is a problem that affects people in a variety of ways. Biologically, individuals may be exposed to drugs that affect mood or may be required to undergo painful medical procedures. Culturally, the childless person may appear deviant to his or her family and friends. In terms of gender roles, if people do not become parents, marital expectations may be disrupted, and career expectations may become more intense (or a job that was never intended to be a career may become more disappointing). Intrapsychically, men and women may feel deeply flawed, cheated, and frustrated. Although most of us who do psychiatric research are trained to adopt some of these perspectives more easily than others, it is important to enlist the help of our colleagues so that we adopt a variety of theoretical perspectives and are able to look at a variety of phenomena in one study—for example, self-esteem, marital satisfaction, psychiatric disorders, and financial and social costs. The help of our statistician colleagues is also essential since study of such a complex issue as psychological response to reproductive interventions must involve many variables, and the appropriate use of multivariate statistical methods is necessary so as not to generate too many spurious significant findings.

The past 10 years have seen remarkable developments in the ability of medical science to assist couples to conceive and bear children. We now have the task of learning from what we have accomplished so far—to find what can be done to make these treatments less stressful for the people undergoing them and to learn for whom the most helpful intervention would be assistance in deciding not to forge ahead to the last possible treatment.

References

Berger DM: Impotence following the discovery of azoospermia. Fertil Steril 34:154–156, 1980a

Berger DM: Couples' reactions to male infertility and donor insemination. Am J Psychiatry 137:1047–1049, 1980b

Bresnick EK: A holistic approach to the treatment of infertility, in Infertility: Medical, Emotional, and Social Considerations. Edited by Mazor MD, Simons HF. New York, Human Sciences Press, 1984, pp 23–35

Bresnick EK, Taymor ML: The role of counselling in infertility. Fertil Steril 32:154–156, 1979

Cella DF, Najavits L: Denial of infertility in patients with Hodgkin's disease. Psychosomatics 27:71, 1986

Collins JA, Wrixon W, Janes LB, et al: Treatment-independent pregnancy among infertile couples. N Engl J Med 309:1201–1244, 1983

Czyba JC, Chevret M: Psychological reactions of couples to artificial insemination with donor sperm. Int J Fertil 24:240–245, 1979

Daniluk JC: Infertility: intrapersonal and interpersonal impact. Fertil Steril 49:982–990, 1988

DeVries K, Degani S, Eibschitz I, et al: The influence of the post-coital test on the sexual function of infertile women. Journal of Psychosomatic Obstetrics and Gynaecology 3:101–106, 1984

Downey J, Yingling S, McKinney M, et al: Mood disorders, psychiatric symptoms, and distress in women presenting for infertility evaluation. Fertil Steril 52:425–432, 1989

Edelmann RJ, Connolly KJ: Psychological aspects of infertility. Br J Med Psychol 59:209–219, 1986

Ellsworth LR, Shain RN: Psychosocial and psychophysiologic aspects of reproduction: the need for improved study design. Fertil Steril 44:449–452, 1985

Erikson E: Childhood and Society. New York, WW Norton, 1950

Erikson E: Life History and the Historical Moment. New York, WW Norton, 1975

Ethics Committee of the American Fertility Society: Ethical Considerations of the New Reproductive Technologies. Birmingham, AL, American Fertility Society, 1986

Freeman EW, Garcia CR, Rickels K: Behavioral and emotional factors: comparisons of anovulatory infertile women with fertile and other infertile women. Fertil Steril 40:195–201, 1983

Garcia CR, Freeman EW, Rickels K, et al: Behavioral and emotional factors and treatment responses in a study of anovulatory infertile women. Fertil Steril 44:478–483, 1985

Hirsch MB, Mosher WD: Characteristics of infertile women in the United States and their use of infertility services. Fertil Steril 47:618–625, 1987

Keye WR: Psychosexual responses to infertility. Clin Obstet Gynecol 27:760–766, 1984

Keye WR, Deneris A, Wilson T, et al: Psychosexual responses to infertility: differences between infertile men and women (abstract). Fertil Steril 36:426, 1981

Lalos A, Lalos O, Jacobsson L, et al: Psychological reactions to the medical investigation and surgical treatment of infertility. Gynecol Obstet Invest 20:209–217, 1985a

Lalos A, Lalos O, Jacobsson L, et al: The psychosocial impact of infertility two years after completed surgical treatment. Acta Obstet Gynecol Scand 64:599–604, 1985b

Lalos A, Lalos O, Jacobsson L, et al: Depression, guilt and isolation among infertile women and their partners. Journal of Psychosomatic Obstetrics and Gynaecology 5:197–206, 1986

Leeton J, Blackwell J: A preliminary psychosocial follow-up of parents and their children conceived by artificial insemination by donor (AID). Clin Reprod Fertil 1:307–310, 1982

Leiblum SR, Kemmann E, Colburn D, et al: Unsuccessful in vitro fertilization: a follow-up study. J In Vitro Fert Embryo Transfer 4:46–50, 1987

Mao K, Wood C: Barriers to treatment of infertility by in-vitro fertilization and embryo transfer. Med J Aust 140:532–533, 1984

Matthews R, Matthews AM: Infertility and involuntary childlessness: the transition to nonparenthood. Journal of Marriage and the Family 48:641–649, 1986

Mazor MD: Emotional reactions to infertility, in Infertility: Medical, Emotional, and Social Considerations. Edited by Mazor MD, Simons HF. New York, Human Services Press, 1984, pp 23–35

McEwan KL, Costello CG, Taylor PG: Adjustment to infertility. J Abnorm Psychol 96:108–116, 1987

Menning BE: The emotional needs of infertile couples. Fertil Steril 34:313–319, 1980

Miall CE: The stigma of involuntary childlessness. Social Problems 33:268–282, 1986

Miller WB: The Personal Meanings of Voluntary and Involuntary Childlessness. Springfield, VA, National Technical Information Service, 1981

Milsom I, Bergman P: A study of parental attitudes after donor insemination. Acta Obstet Gynecol Scand 61:125–128, 1982

Morse C, Dennerstein L: Infertile couples entering an in vitro fertilization programme: a preliminary survey. Journal of Psychosomatic Obstetrics and Gynaecology 4:207–219, 1985

Mushin DN, Barreda-Hanson MC, Spensley JC: In vitro fertilization children: early psychosocial development. J In Vitro Fert Embryo Transfer 3:247–252, 1986

Parker PJ: Motivations of surrogate mothers: initial findings. Am J Psychiatry 140:117–118, 1983

Paulson JD, Harrmann BS, Salerno RL, et al: An investigation of the relationship between emotional maladjustment and infertility. Fertil Steril 49:258–262, 1988

Reame NE: Maternal adaptation and psychologic responses to a surrogate pregnancy (abstract). Presented at the 43rd annual meeting of the American Fertility Society, Reno, NV, 1987

Rosenfeld DL, Mitchell E: Treating the emotional aspects of infertility: counselling services in an infertility clinic. Am J Obstet Gynecol 135:177–180, 1979

Snarey J, Son L, Kuehne VS, et al: The role of parenting in men's psychosocial development: a longitudinal study of early adulthood infertility and midlife generativity. Developmental Psychology 23:593–603, 1987

Sokoloff BZ: Alternative methods of reproduction: effects on the child. Clin Pediatr (Phila) 26:11–17, 1987

Spensley JC, Mushin D, Barreda-Hanson M: The children of IVF pregnancies: a cohort study. Aust Paediatr J 22:285–289, 1986

Speroff L, Glass RH, Kase NG: Clinical Gynecologic Endocrinology and Infertility. Baltimore, MD, Williams & Wilkins, 1983

Valentine DP: Psychological impact of infertility: identifying needs and issues. Soc Work Health Care 11:61–69, 1986

DATE DUE

JUN 2 2 1992		
JE 3 '92	JAN 1 0 1997	
	JAN 0 6 1997	
MAR 1 3 1994		
MAR 1 6		
MAY 2 4 1995		
JUN 1 4 1995		
JUN 0 1 1995		
NOV 0 7 1996		
JAN 1 4 2004		
5/5/06		

DEMCO 38-297